Pregnancy Week by Week

Pregnancy Book For First Time Moms

The 3 Trimesters of Pregnancy
1 Week Pregnant – 40 Weeks Pregnant

By Babette Lansing

Disclaimer

Published by Babette Lansing
Venus Epubs
www.whattoknowaboutpregnancy.co

ISBN-13:978-1481808675
ISBN-10:1481808672

Printed in the United States of America.

About The Author

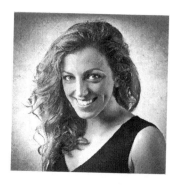

Babette Lansing is the up-and-coming author/illustrator of several beautifully illustrated books for young children. Her life-long love of children started early, as she is the eldest of six brothers and sisters.

She was inspired to write about pregnancy and childbirth after she realized that the majority of books on these topics are lengthy and time-consuming to read. As we all know, most expectant and new mothers are far too busy to read 200+ pages at any given time. This is why she has boiled down the relevant information into a manuscript that is clearly subdivided into easy-to-read portions.

Babette Lansing will tell you that being a mother is her life's greatest happiness. She hopes that you, as the reader, will enjoy this book as much as she enjoyed writing it.

To visit Babette Lansing's pregnancy and childcare website, go to and see all her books:

WhatToKnowAboutPregnancy.co

To visit Babette Lansing's children's book website, go to:

BooksOnlineForKids.info

Table Of Contents

The Third Semester

Introduction

This book will take you week by week through all 3 trimesters of pregnancy and provide you with vital information about what is happening inside your body and the development of your unborn child.

The information provided by this book has been prepared for general information, reference, and educational purposes only; it is not intended to take the place of professional medical advice.

You, as the reader, should not act upon any advice contained in this book without first consulting your primary care provider.

Call 911 or contact your doctor if you are experiencing a medical emergency.

Ask your OB/GYN if you need further information or have any concerns.

Congratulations on your soon-to-be little one!
I hope you will enjoy my book.

Babette Lansing

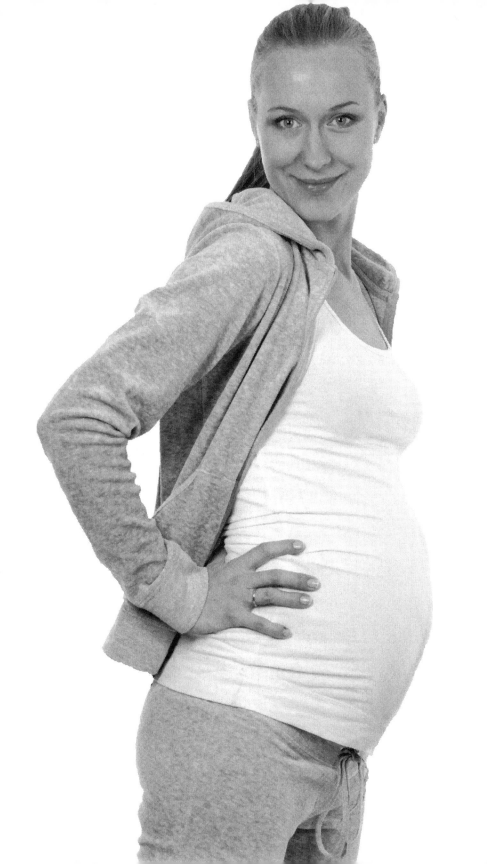

The First Trimester

1 Week Pregnant – 13 Weeks Pregnant

A week-by-week pregnancy calendar is a must-have for any pregnant woman, especially if she is expecting her first child. Knowing what is happening inside you during pregnancy can spare you anxiety and help you solve problems that may arise throughout the course of your pregnancy. Please consult your OB/GYN if you need further information or have any concerns whatsoever...

The First Trimester of Pregnancy
is a period of great changes. Emotionally, these are the most difficult weeks of your pregnancy. Your thoughts are focused on your body, and you may feel isolated from the rest of the world. You are very introverted during this period, and your partner may find you absentminded and distractible. Just remember, this too shall pass. These emotional changes are very normal, and learning about your bodily changes will help you to better understand your condition.

Keep reading to find out what is going on inside your body week by week:

First Week of Pregnancy

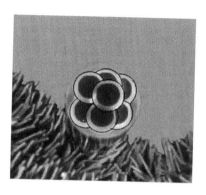

Few things in life bring as much joy as the successful conception of a baby. The sheer knowledge that you are expecting is empowering and wonderful. However, since it is calculated based upon gestational age, the first week of pregnancy is usually a mystery. This is the time when the egg and sperm meet, and a woman may not be aware that she is pregnant for several more weeks.

If you are anticipating pregnancy, you must adjust to new habits and prepare for upcoming changes. During this stage, you may experience the mixed emotions of joy, fear, and excitement. A woman, especially if she is a first-time mom, must prepare her heart and mind for the experience ahead of her. During the first week of pregnancy, the "baby" is not yet a baby. The fetus is still preparing to be formed, making this the most crucial aspect of the entire pregnancy process.

Physical Changes

During the first two weeks of the first trimester, pregnancy can-not be absolutely confirmed. Therefore, you will not know for a while whether or not conception was successful. In terms of physical changes, these two weeks are probably the easiest part of any pregnancy. Emotionally, however, waiting for results can be stressful, especially if a woman is desperate for a child.

Though you may not be readily aware of whether or not you are pregnant, speculations can be made if you keep careful record of your menstrual cycle. Obstetricians and midwives typically use the first day of the last menstrual period to calcu-late the gestational age of the baby.

Physical changes may not be apparent yet at this stage, but you still need to treat your body with utmost care. Whether you are actually expecting a baby or not, it is best to put an end to unhealthy habits such as smoking, drinking alcoholic beverages, and going to bed late.

It would also be advisable to take prenatal vitamins such as folic acid. This is a kind of Vitamin B that prevents brain and neural-tube defects in the unborn baby. It is best to start taking folic acid early in a pregnancy.
Avoid harmful exposure X-rays and radiation while awaiting results. It is always best to play it safe.

Mental and Emotional Preparation

The first week of pregnancy is a good time to prepare mentally and emotionally for the months ahead. Steel yourself for cramps, morning sickness, back pain, and other uncomfortable pregnancy symptoms.

If you are still unaware of the fact that you are pregnant, emotional upheaval may occur. Some women experience emotional confusion because they are not sure whether or not they are ready to have a baby. These women may benefit from support groups that will assist in preparing them mentally and emotionally. Every pregnant woman needs to accept her pregnancy with all her heart in order to have a healthy pregnancy experience.

The Baby

According to the gestational-age method, the first week of pregnancy begins the first day of a woman's last menstrual period. Conception has not yet occurred, but significant changes begin to take place. During this time, the uterine lining is shed and the fertilized ovum is released. The egg and the sperm will then meet, and the egg will multiply its cells as it begins its journey to the uterus.

Second Week of Pregnancy

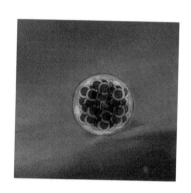

The second week of pregnancy is still too early for a woman to feel changes in her body. It is for the sake of convenience that doctors refer to this period as the second week of pregnancy; however, the fact is that a woman at this stage is still not pregnant in the true sense of the word. The egg has not actually been fertilized yet; actual fertilization will not occur until the end of this week.

Changes within the Body

There are changes taking place within the body during this period, but because these are slow and take place deep within the body, they generally go unnoticed by the expectant mother. The first obvious change is that the lining of the uterus begins to develop in preparation for the pregnancy. The uterus starts building reserves, which will provide nourishment to the baby throughout the pregnancy. At the same time, the body produces high levels of FSH (follicle stimulating hormone), which acts as a stimulator and literally incites the egg to mature.

By the end of week two a woman will have reached the middle of her menstruation cycle, provided she has a regular 28-day cycle. At this time, ovulation occurs, and FSH levels in the blood are high. A mature egg is released by the ovary, moves into the Fallopian tube, and begins traveling toward the uterus. Unprotected sexual intercourse during this phase can easily result in a pregnancy.

When a man ejaculates inside a woman's vagina, he releases millions of microscopic sperms, invisible to the unaided human eye. The sperms swim through the vagina in the direction of the Fallopian tube. Only a few hundred of them actually reach the

Fallopian tube, where the mature egg that was released by the ovary is present. It takes only one sperm penetrating an egg for fertilization to occur. Once the egg is fertilized, the woman becomes pregnant.

Special Care throughout the Second Week

This is the right time to implement lifestyle changes in anticipation of impending pregnancy. Quit smoking and give up alcohol as well, as these could hamper the baby's growth. Doctors recommend that women cut down on caffeine intake and concentrate on proper eating habits. (Read more about caffeine intake in the chapter: "Ninth Week of Pregnancy")

A pregnant woman must watch what she eats. A diet rich in fresh vegetables, fruits, and whole grains is recommended by doctors. Adding nuts, low-fat dairy, and meat products to the diet will provide nutrition to both the mother and the tiny embryo that will be ready for implanting by the end of the second week. These foods will boost the pregnant woman's energy levels, as well as help her cope with pregnancy-related symptoms. Eating smaller meals more frequently is a beneficial practice. The second week of pregnancy is also the right time to implement a daily exercise routine that can be used throughout pregnancy.

By three weeks, a woman is definitely pregnant. At this stage, the egg has been fertilized and has firmly implanted itself in the lining of the womb. Although it is still too early to begin seeing changes in the body, the baby inside is most certainly developing rapidly. A woman at three weeks may not feel any of the symptoms of pregnancy yet, but the baby she has conceived is already taking shape.

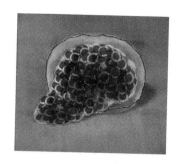

Growth of the Baby

Conception is such a wondrous gift of nature that a woman must understand how it happens. The egg is released and fertilized within the first two weeks of pregnancy, at which point the egg cells begin to divide quickly. Within thirty hours of fertilization, the egg has divided in two. The cells keep doubling until there are a total of 64 cells. While cell division is in progress, the fertilized egg is also moving along the Fallopian tube toward the uterus. By the time it reaches the uterus, the egg is a cluster of divided cells that resemble a mulberry. The fertilized egg at this stage is called a morula.

The tiny, fluid-filled morula further divides in two and is then referred to as a blastocyst. By the end of the third week, the blastocyst has divided as well and adheres itself to the inner wall of the uterus, also known as the endometrium. One portion of the blastocyst forms a placenta, and the other begins its journey toward becoming a baby. At this point, the baby is still an embryo and has not yet become a fetus. The placenta is the embryo's lifeline and will continue to be so until it is born. The placenta provides the growing embryo with vital nutrients and helps it to excrete its waste.

Self-Care during this Period

At three weeks pregnant, it is essential that a woman take utmost care of her diet and nutrition. There are some minerals, vitamins, and nutrients that are vital for the proper growth of a baby. The pregnant woman needs to ensure that her diet is well-balanced so that she will receive adequate amounts of the required nutrients.

Doctors prescribe folic acid, iron capsules, and calcium tablets during this period and all throughout pregnancy. Folic acid is especially important to the prevention of defects in the embryo that can occur during early pregnancy. Calcium is required for the baby's bones and teeth.

A pregnant woman needs to keep her calcium intake high so that there is adequate supply of the mineral for the baby's growth. Iron supplements are also essential during this time, as they help provide the baby's continual demand for blood. Protein is vital for proper tissue development.

Diet

A pregnant woman must include plenty of greens, vegetables, and fruits in her diet in order to provide herself and her unborn baby with necessary nutrients. In addition, low-fat dairy products must also be consumed for the calcium they will provide. Red meat, leafy green vegetables, eggs, and legumes are all good sources of iron. Red meat and eggs are also rich in protein. A balanced diet with all of these foods should provide a pregnant woman with every nutrient necessary for a healthy baby and a healthy pregnancy.

Congratulations! You are four weeks pregnant. NOW WHAT? The best thing about being four weeks pregnant is that you have been pregnant for nearly a month and have hardly even known it. In terms of hormonal fluctuations and bodily changes, this is the best it will get for a while. And only eight months from now, you will be holding your little one snug in your arms!

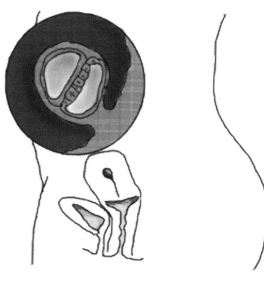

What Exactly is Going on with Your Baby at Four Weeks Pregnant?

The ball of cells that will develop into your baby in just a few short weeks is no bigger than a poppy seed. Now that the egg has completed its journey from the Fallopian tube to the uterus, the blastocyst will split in two. Half will form into the embryo, while the other half begins its specialization into the placenta. The embryo is further divided into three parts; the endoderm, mesoderm, and ectoderm. The endoderm, which is the internal layer, will develop into the digestive system, liver, and lungs of your baby. The mesoderm, or middle layer, is slated to become your baby's heart, sex organs, bones, kidneys, and muscles. Finally, the ectoderm, or outer layer, will specialize into the nervous system, hair, skin, and eyes of your baby.

What is Going On with Your Body
at Four Weeks Pregnant?

You have probably used a least five at-home pregnancy tests just to see the word "pregnant" pop up on the screen. This is an exciting time that will bring with it a number of changes. Your breasts will likely be noticeably heavy and tender (especially the nipples), much like they are around the time of your period, only magnified. This is due to an increase in estrogen and progesterone, preparing your breasts to feed your baby in a few short months.

Progesterone will also slow down your digestion in order to allow your body to redirect as many nutrients as possible to the baby as food travels through your body. This may result in feelings of bloatedness and an increased sensation of fullness. Morning sickness, if you are going to have it, will not begin for another 1-2 weeks, so enjoy this time of relatively symptom-free pregnancy while it lasts. Emotionally, you probably have not even begun to process what is going on, but do not worry. You have another 36 weeks to become acclimated to the new life inside of you and all that it implies.

You might think that four weeks pregnant is too early for any sort of planning, but you can begin taking baby steps to prepare yourself for the weeks to come. Ask around to find an OB/GYN that is highly recommended in your area. Finding a competent one is crucial, as you will be seeing a LOT of this professional as your pregnancy progresses.

Fifth Week of Pregnancy

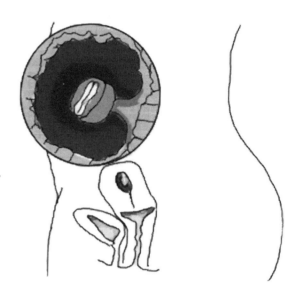

Now that you are five weeks pregnant, you have officially entered the second month of your pregnancy. Congratulations!

What is Going on with Your Baby at Five Weeks Pregnant?

Your baby is now about the size of an orange seed and resembles a tiny tadpole, complete with tail. The circulatory system, which circulates blood throughout the body, is the first part of the baby to begin functioning. This means that you may see a tiny beating heart on an early ultrasound sometime in the next few weeks. Another part that is forming at this time is the neural tube, which will eventually become the baby's brain and spinal cord.

What is Going on with Your Body at Five Weeks Pregnant?

Week five is pivotal in many ways, as early pregnancy symptoms seem to kick in around this point. Morning sickness, which affects nearly half of pregnant women, may rear its ugly head during this week. Morning sickness is a misnomer, as the queasy feelings can persist all day long, coming and going in waves that leave you exhausted. You may be ravenously hungry, but absolutely nothing looks even remotely appealing to you. This is completely normal, and the good news is, most morning-sickness sufferers will feel markedly different by week thirteen.

The bad news is, this is only week five. Hang in there! You can make it! Some tips to help you get through morning sickness are to make sure to nibble on small meals throughout the day-- whenever you do not feel queasy, grab something that appeals to you. For many women, this tends to be comfort food, such as macaroni and cheese. Strong odors and tastes are an enemy during this time, even previous favorites such as garlic or soy sauce. Do your best to avoid foods that are especially pungent. Sipping on ginger-ale has been shown to have stomach-settling effects, as has drinking a cup of ginger-laced tea.

Because the baby's neural tube is developing this week, it is especially important to be diligent with taking your prenatal vitamin supplement. Prenatal supplements that contain 400 micrograms of Folic acid have been shown to reduce the risks of neural-related diseases such as spina bifida by nearly 50%. If even swallowing the pill makes you sick, try taking it in the evening, when the hormone levels that cause morning sickness may be lower.

In addition to nausea, frequent urination and extreme fatigue are very common. Again, these symptoms will gradually diminish as you near your second trimester; in the meantime, you must tough it out as best you can. Take naps (if you are able) and decrease your commitments. It is important to listen to your body and not overtax yourself. Moderate exercise, surprisingly enough, will go a long way toward boosting your energy level, as the "endorphin high" that comes from aerobic exercise will somewhat counteract feelings of lassitude. At this stage o in your pregnancy, it is all right to continue with your regular exercise regimen, but please speak with your OB/GYN if you have any concerns.

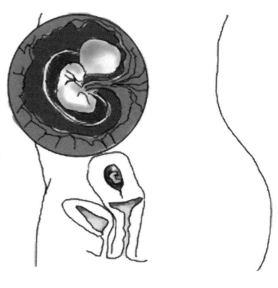

Now that you are six weeks pregnant, you may be struggling to adjust to an unfamiliar lifestyle. Morning sickness most likely began last week, leaving you little time to acclimate your body to the demanding task of keeping abreast of those waves of nausea. Give yourself a daily pep talk. You will pull through!

What is Going On with Your Baby at Six Weeks Pregnant?

Though your baby is only about the size of a nail-head at this point, there are many exciting developments this week. For starters, your baby may already have your nose, as this is the week that baby's facial structure, including jaw, chin, eyes, ears, and nose, begin to take shape. Internally, your baby's heart, liver, and lungs are developing, and the heart is beating at a rate of 80 beats per minute.

What is Going On with Your Body at Six Weeks Pregnant?

These are still the early days; there is no need to start maternity-clothes shopping just yet--believe me, you will have more than enough time to model that maternity couture over the coming months! Enjoy your regular clothes as much as possible right now, although you may need to make some accommodations, such as selecting looser-fitting articles of non-maternity clothing.

During week six, you may notice a higher frequency of urination due to the increase of blood flow to your pelvic area, making your kidneys much more efficient in filtration. Your uterus is also starting to put pressure on your bladder. Do not stop drinking water in an attempt to curb frequent urination, and go to the bathroom when the urge strikes, otherwise you may find your-self with a bladder infection.

In addition to frequent urination, your constant companions this week will be bloating, fatigue, and low-level nausea. Your sense of smell will be heightened, which will most likely increase your nausea. Hang in there--studies have shown that women who ex-perience morning sickness are less likely to miscarry than those who do not. You may notice changes in your breasts; besides increased the tenderness and fullness, your areolas (the skin around the nipples) may darken, creating a "bulls-eye" on your chest for your soon-to-be little nursling.

This week, you will most likely be introduced to new symptoms that may last until the very end of your pregnancy--heartburn. Don't take antacids especially Tums. Heartburn is a symptom that indicates poor digestion and the presence of acid reflux - taking the tablets only makes it worse. Taking antacids will reduce stomach acid and low stomach acid can lead to a leaky gut which causes other major issues.

Eating fermented foods, lifestyle changes eating 5 or 6 small meals a day, avoiding spicy or greasy food, and not lying down for 1 hour after eating will remedy the problem. Also eating yo-gurt and drinking milk.

Spotting in early pregnancy is quite common, but it can under-standably cause concern. Contact your OB/GYN if you have any worries.

Now that you are seven weeks pregnant, you are closing in on the end of your second month. Early pregnancy symptoms--such as nausea, heartburn, indigestion, and fatigue--are still going strong. But what else is happening inside your body?

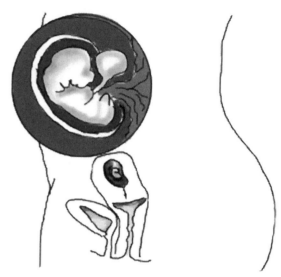

What to Expect From Your Baby at Seven Weeks Pregnant

Your baby is still considered an embryo at this stage, and still has a tiny tail, but the big news this week is that baby's hands and feet are emerging from that tiny little body (now about the size of a blueberry). They look a lot like paddles at this stage, but soon enough will be completely formed. Your baby has doubled in size in just one week---no wonder you are fatigued! In addition, your baby's eyelid folds now partially cover his or her eyes, which already are somewhat colored. Both hemispheres of baby's brain are growing, and the liver is creating red blood cells until the bone marrow is ready to take over this job. There is an appendix, and a pancreas, which will soon be producing insulin to aid in digestion. The umbilical cord has now formed distinct blood vessels that carry oxygen and nutrients to and from the tiny baby.

At seven weeks pregnant, you may be experiencing extreme mood swings--you may go from being wildly elated to sobbing in the span of one sappy TV commercial. These intense emotional surges are normal, and should completely dissipate after you have given birth.

Bloating and fatigue will be still going strong; give yourself a break as often as possible, and try to avoid excess salt, which will increase bloating. Keep up your exercise regimen, as this will help you maintain strength and flexibility during the course of your pregnancy. Think of pregnancy as training for a marathon-keeping yourself goal-oriented will greatly increase your chances of having a complication-free birth. Exercise will also help you de-stress, and may even increase the appetite that morning sickness has stolen from you.

Energize yourself with small snacks that pair a protein with a complex carbohydrate--such as cheese and crackers or peanut butter on toast. This will give you a boost of energy while still being gentle on your upset stomach.

Within the next week or so, you should schedule your first appointment with your OB/GYN. This will be an important appointment, as your chosen health professional will review your medical history, give you your due date (you may already know it), and go over any concerns that you may have regarding your pregnancy. Be prepared by knowing the date of your last period, the genetic and medical history of you and your partner, and the name of any medications that you are currently taking. Jot down any questions you may have; there is no reason to be shy, and there is no such thing as a stupid question. As the one who is pregnant, you may have insights into your symptoms that your doctors are not privy to, so listen to your body and ask away!

Eighth Week of Pregnancy

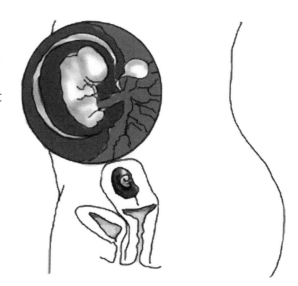

You are now two months pregnant--in just a few short weeks, you will be out of the first trimester and into the smooth sailing that is the second trimester. So, what can you expect this week?

Your Baby at Eight Weeks Pregnant: What to Expect

At eight weeks, your baby is about the size of a kidney bean. The tail is nearly gone, and the eyelids are almost fully formed. There are now breathing tubes extending from the throat to the developing lungs, although your baby will not take a first breath until after the birth, as babies continue to receive oxygen via the placenta for the duration of the pregnancy. In the brain, nerve cells are forming early pathways, and branching out to connect to one another. The external genitalia are not quite developed enough to see whether your baby will be a girl or a boy, but very soon you will be able to find out. Baby is constantly moving around, though you will not be able to feel those first flutters for another ten weeks or so.

Your Body at Eight Weeks Pregnant: What to Expect

Your breasts will continue their alarming rate of growth all throughout your pregnancy. Most women go up anywhere from one to two cup sizes, making pregnancy one of the first times that some women's "cups runneth over". Get fitted for a new bra as soon as you can--you want to ensure that your enlarging breasts have proper support. You may want to go ahead and invest in a nursing bra with underwire--you will get double use out of it, both during your pregnancy and during your nursing period.

Nursing bras need not be frumpy; there are plenty of lovely, lace-embellished ones out there that will get the job done. Look for wide, comfortable straps, easy one-handed cup closure release, and a layer of padding that will absorb any leakage that gets past your nursing pad. Glamorous, no? Even if you are not planning on breast feeding, your breasts will not figure this out until a week or so postpartum; you will need to have a supportive bra on hand that will work during the engorgement period.

Around eight weeks, many couples begin to tell their families their exciting news. You may wish to hold off until the first trimester is over, or tell only those whom you feel would support you in the tragic event of a miscarriage. There is no need to spend nights agonizing over whether you will lose the baby, as you are probably sleep-deprived enough due to frequent urination. Most pregnancies will continue, and only those in which the baby truly would not have had a chance outside your body will result in a miscarriage. Try not to live in fear, but educate yourself about the risks and responsibilities that you are facing. It goes without saying that cigarette smoking and alcohol consumption should NOT be indulged in during pregnancy. Speak with your OB/GYN regarding other dietary and lifestyle restrictions, just to be sure that you are maintaining the healthiest possible environment for you precious cargo.

Ninth Week of Pregnancy

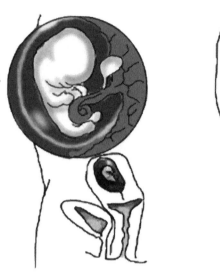

Now that you are nine weeks pregnant, you are well into your first trimester. For the very first time, you may be accepting the fact that you are indeed pregnant.

What is Going On with Your Baby at Nine Weeks Pregnant?

At nine weeks gestational age, your baby is the size of a grape--about an inch long--and weighs just a fraction of an ounce. All of the essential body parts are present and accounted for, though they will still undergo some fine-tuning during the months ahead. Baby has moved out of the embryonic stage, and the tail is now completely gone. Baby looks nearly human, and is considered a full-fledged fetus. The heart has finished dividing into four chambers, and the valves are beginning to form, along with baby's first set of teeth, which are beginning to bud underneath the gums. External sex organs are present, but hold off on painting the nursery just yet--they will be indistinguishable for another few weeks. By week nine, baby has fully formed eyes, but the lids are fused shut and will not open until around 27 weeks. Tiny earlobes are present, and other facial features are becoming more and more distinct. The placenta is fully developed, and begins to take over the critical job of producing hormones. Now that baby's physiology is basically in place, next week will be a time of rapid weight gain.

What is Going On with Your Body at Nine Weeks Pregnant?

Morning sickness, nausea, fatigue, and heartburn are still going strong at nine weeks pregnant. If you are working, and were not planning to spill the beans until the first trimester is over, you may want to revise that plan in order to let your boss know why you are always bolting out of the conference room when someone brings in an egg-salad sandwich. Telling just one or two people will give you a support system, and will help make the workplace bearable during this difficult time.

Extreme mood swings also come with the territory around this time, and may be aggravated by the near constant state of exhaustion that you are stumbling around in--between the crushing fatigue and the constant nighttime interruptions as you empty your bladder yet again, you are just not getting much sleep these days. Cheer up! Once your newborn arrives, you will have already made it through nine months of "sleep deprivation boot camp", and should be primed to rock the mommy role.

Caffeine might be consumed by pregnant women in moderation but be careful! 300 mg caffeine or less is OK. Dr. Daniel Amen who is a clinical neuroscientist, brain imaging expert, and clinical psychiatrist in his book 2012 - "Change Your Brain, Change Your Life" recommends pregnant women to watch how their body responds to caffeine and keep it to a minimum. There have been studies done that indicate caffeine interferes with fertility, causes low birth weight, associated with premature births. There have been some positive outcomes from other studies as well. But being careful is an important consideration according to Dr. Amen.

Week nine is normally the week in which you will head to the OB/GYN for that first meeting, so have your medical history, list of medications, and any questions or concerns prepared before you head off to that first exciting appointment.

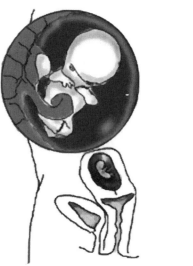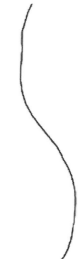

Well done! You have made it to ten weeks! In just four more weeks, you will leave the first trimester behind you and with it, many of those uncomfortable symptoms you have been dealing with – such as morning sickness, fatigue, and nausea.

What is Going On with Your Baby at Ten Weeks Pregnant?

At ten weeks, baby is now about the size of a prune--a little over an inch from crown to rump. Now that the most critical portion of development is completed, baby's tissues and organs begin to rapidly grow and mature. This week, baby begins to swallow fluid, and kick, kick, kick, though you will not feel it for another ten weeks or so. The vital organs, including kidneys, intestines, liver, and brain, are fully formed and beginning to function; although there are continued developments ahead, the majority have already taken place. The yolk sac is disappearing; its red-blood-cell-manufacturing role is diminishing, and being assumed by the liver. Tiny finger- and toenails are forming, and baby is coated with downy hair. Baby's limbs can bend now, and the feet may be long enough to meet in front of the body. The spine is visible through translucent skin, and spinal nerves are beginning to form. At this stage, baby's head is more than half the length of the body, and bulges temporarily with the developing brain.

What is Going On with Your Body
at Ten Weeks Pregnant?

Same old, same old this week--your dear friends nausea, fatigue, and maybe heartburn too are still making you uncomfortable. The good news is, at ten weeks pregnant, especially if you are slim to begin with or if this is not your first pregnancy, you may begin to see the tiniest of bulges below your navel. This week may be time for you to start rethinking your wardrobe, as your pants may be getting harder to button.

You can buy yourself some time by placing a hair elastic through the button hole and looping it around the button, or investing in a belly band--a wide, stretchy band of fabric which you can wear over your jeans to hide the fact that they are no longer button-ing, and in later weeks, cover your burgeoning belly from shirts which are suddenly too short. Belly bands are a good investment even for the postpartum period; they can be worn under a shirt to provide some privacy for nursing--simply lift your top shirt and nurse, leaving your belly covered by the band.

If your first prenatal appointment was scheduled this week, you may be lucky enough to hear your baby's heartbeat with the Doppler--a hand-held instrument that is completely non-inva-sive, and picks up your baby's heartbeat through the skin of your belly. There is absolutely no sound like it in the world, and you may become teary at the knowledge that there is, in fact, a little person inside of you. Once the heartbeat is found, and it appears to be strong, the relative risk of miscarriage drops to an even lower percentage. Waiting to share your good news until after you hear the baby's heartbeat is almost always a safe bet.

Eleventh Week of Pregnancy

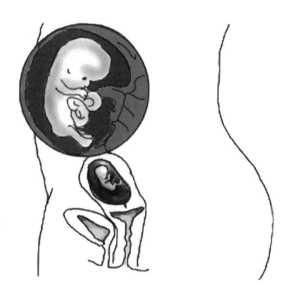

Now that you are eleven weeks pregnant, you are in the last few weeks of your first trimester and probably excited to put it behind you. What is happening with your baby and your body this week?

What is Happening with Your Baby at Eleven Weeks Pregnant?

Baby is now about the size of a lime, or about 2 inches long from crown to toes. Baby now looks distinctly human, down to its perfectly formed ears, nostrils, and tongue and hard palate inside the mouth. Baby also has distinct toes and fingers with no more webbing between them. Perfectly distinct nipples can be found on both male and female embryos, and hair follicles have been formed on the head, nearly ready to start growing hair. Baby's skin is still translucent, but other than that, he or she is completely recognizable as a human.

What is Happening with Your Body at Eleven Weeks Pregnant?

Your morning sickness may be (finally!) starting to ease up, but do not despair—you will have a new set of troubles to contend with now that your appetite is back, namely constipation and flatulence. Because progesterone slows your digestive muscles to enable full assimilation of all possible nutrients and calories, you may be struggling to keep yourself regular.

Try to increase your fiber intake, as well as your water intake; both of these will aid significantly in maintaining regularity. Continue with your exercise program, as this has also been shown to help ease constipation.

Around eleven weeks, you may also become light-headed and may even faint, as your body is not yet producing enough blood to keep up with your expanding circulatory system. However, this symptom is very short-lived and may be alleviated by keeping your blood sugar stable with healthy snacking.

Sometime between eleven and thirteen weeks, your doctor may schedule a series of tests known as first trimester screening. This completely safe, non-invasive (for the baby) series of tests involves a maternal blood screen, as well as an early ultrasound. Doctors can use the results from the scan and the test to determine risk levels for disorders such as Down's Syndrome and Trisomy-18.

A portion of the test, called the nuchal translucency test, measures the skin fold at the back of baby's neck. This measurement is a determinant for other conditions such as cardiac abnormalities.

What should you do if the results from these tests are less than reassuring? First of all, do not panic! These tests are by no means 100% definitive--they measure probabilities, not actualities. Even if your odds are higher than normal, there is still a very good chance that there will be nothing at all wrong with your baby. If there is a red flag, there are still options for further, more invasive testing that may tell you more about what you and your partner should expect.

Twelve weeks have quickly gone by, and you are just about into your second trimester. Only a little over 2/3 of the way to go! You may still be able to easily camouflage your "delicate condition," or you may be sporting a tiny baby bump, especially if this is not your first pregnancy. What can you expect this week?

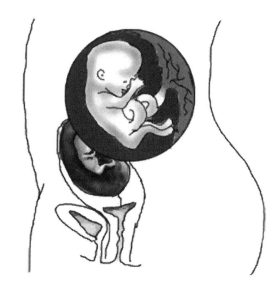

What is Going On with Your Baby at Twelve Weeks Pregnant?

The biggest change this week is the development of your baby's reflexes. The fingers open and close, the toes clench, and the mouth makes sucking movements. If you poke the side of your abdomen, baby will squirm in response, though he or she is still too small for you to be able to feel it; the baby is still about two inches long, only about the size of a lime. At twelve weeks, baby's nerve cells are multiplying rapidly, and synapses are firing inside its brain. Baby looks unquestionably human at this point—his or her eyes have moved to the front of the face, and the ears are positioned perfectly on the side of the head.

What is Going On with Your Body at Twelve Weeks Pregnant?

Your morning sickness will (finally!) be abating somewhat, though some women are not in the clear until fourteen weeks.

For some unlucky women, feelings of nausea will return late in the third trimester, but that is still far enough away that it should not be a concern right now.

Your uterus has risen and grown to the point where your health-care provider can feel the top of it, called the fundus, low in your abdomen, right above your pubic bone. You are probably in that strange no-man's land between fitting into some of your looser clothing and wishing you had some maternity pants about now. If you have not yet invested in a belly band, now is the time. Remember that maternity clothing does not have to be frumpy; there are beautiful, flattering styles out there for every stage of pregnancy. Buy a few key pieces, and do not forget to accessorize. If you cannot justify a whole-new wardrobe that will last only nine months, ask your friends if you can borrow some of their old maternity clothes.

Maybe heartburn will still be a concern at this point. You are most likely to notice its intensity in the evening hours, or when you lie down for the night. This is completely normal and does not signify anything to be concerned about. Talk to your OB/GYN and see if there is prescription of antacids he or she can recommend if you can't remedy the problem the way I recommended. Spotting is also fairly common during this period, especially immediately after intercourse. Because your cervix is more heavily vascularized due to the increase in blood flow to your pelvis, it is more likely to bleed after sex. Unless there is heavy bleeding, or you see any clots larger than a dime, there is no cause for concern.

Thirteenth Week of Pregnancy

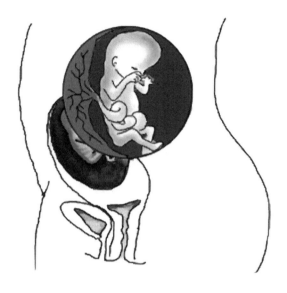

This is it! The last week of your first trimester! At this point in your pregnancy, you probably feel that it cannot go by fast enough. Fortunately, it should be smooth sailing for the next few months; the second trimester is a bit like the eye of a hurricane, in that many of the problems that plague a pregnant woman in the first trimester, and the impending birth that looms in the third trimester, are nowhere to be found. The only things going on in the next few months are appointments, screening tests, and of course, the big ultrasound around eighteen weeks. Let us take a look at what is happening to you and your baby in your thirteenth week.

What is Going On with Your Baby at Thirteen Weeks Pregnant?

Your baby is now ready for a life of crime--as fingerprints have finally formed on his or her tiny fingertips! Baby's skin is still translucent, and the veins and organs are clearly visible. Baby's body, formerly less than half of the total length, is starting to catch up with the head, which is now only one-third of baby's body length. If your baby is a girl, your future grand-babies are already possibilities! At thirteen weeks, baby girls have several million eggs in their ovaries. Baby is about three inches long, (about the size of a medium shrimp), and weighs about one ounce.

What is Going On with Your Body at Thirteen Weeks Pregnant?

Good news, good news, and more good news about your body at thirteen weeks pregnant! For starters, that pesky morning sickness has probably just about run its course, restoring you to your former food-loving ways. Ditto on the fatigue, as many women experience a surge of energy that lasts until the last few weeks of pregnancy.

Now is the time to get things done! You will be utterly amazed at what a pregnant woman can accomplish in just a few short weeks--once the fainting, puking, and falling asleep randomly is behind her, that is! More good news for this week is that your libido may be starting to return. This is partly due to the continued increase of blood flow to your pelvic region, keeping you semi-engorged much of the time, especially when you are up and walking about. You may find that your sex life with your partner takes a huge leap forward; many women who previously struggled to achieve climax now suddenly find that it is no longer an issue, due to increased sensitivity.

Now for some not-so-great news: leucorrhea, a whitish vaginal discharge that protects against infection, is being produced in larger quantities. Not to worry; just stock up on panty-liners and you should be good to go.

By now your OB/GYN should have the results back from your first trimester screen, and will more than likely go over them with you at your next appointment, which should be soon. If you were unable to hear the fetal heartbeat during your first appointment, you should definitely be able to hear it by now. Enjoy these precious moments of your pregnancy!

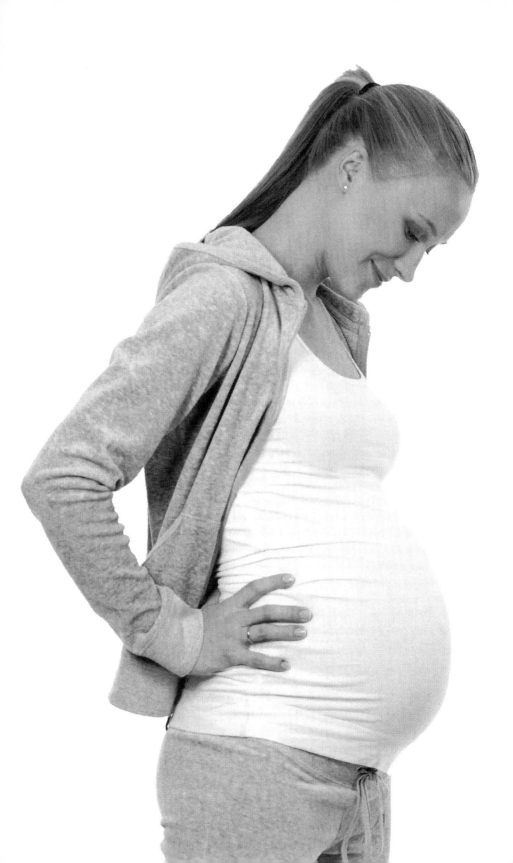

The Second Trimester

14 Week Pregnant – 26 Weeks Pregnant

The second trimester is a more balanced period for most women than either the first or third trimesters, but some still experience morning sickness and other physical symptoms such as extreme exhaustion. During weeks 20 – 24, you will start to feel your baby kicking, making you more aware than ever that you are eating, sleeping, and living for two.

Keep reading to find out what is going on inside your body week by week:

Welcome to the first week of your second trimester, the so-called "honeymoon phase" of pregnancy. Compared to the first and last trimesters, this trimester is a breeze! What can you expect this week?

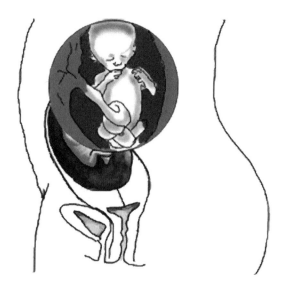

What is Going On with Your Baby at Fourteen Weeks Pregnant?

Due to newly developed brain impulses, baby can now form expressions on its teeny-tiny face, including squinting, frowning, and sucking its thumb. Baby's kidneys are producing urine, which is released into the amniotic fluid. Baby measures about 3.5 inches from top to bottom, about the size of a lemon, and weighs in around 1.5 ounces. Its body is finally outpacing the growth of its head, making its proportions more recognizable. This week, baby will develop a distinct neck, and arms will become proportionate to the rest of the body. Baby is covered with a downy hair called lanugo, which protects its skin from the water bath where it resides. Internally, baby's liver starts to manufacture bile, and the spleen aids in the production of red blood cells. Baby is extremely active in its home--punching, kicking, and doing somersaults, none of which you will be able to feel for a few more weeks.

What is Going On with Your Body at Fourteen Weeks Pregnant?

Your energy is likely on the upswing once again, and your morning sickness is probably all but gone. Your breasts may be less tender than before (though still larger than normal), and best of all, fourteen weeks marks a huge drop in the risk of miscarriage, making fourteen weeks a great time to begin letting people know your happy news.

The fundus (top of your uterus) is now beginning to protrude above your pubic bone, signifying the beginnings of that cute baby bump. Most women who are pregnant for the first time notice a definite bulge that can no longer be attributed to the effects of bloating. Maternity clothes are now a necessity--especially pants. You may be able to get away with your normal tops for a few more weeks, especially if they are longer tops.

There are several kinds of maternity pants, ranging from trousers to jeans and capris, and you will probably want several pairs of each, depending on which seasons your pregnancy spans. Maternity clothing follows pre-pregnancy sizing, taking a lot of the guesswork out of purchasing. "Under the belly" demi-panels may be most comfortable at this early phase, as you will not be able to fill the "full panel" jeans for quite some time.

As far as weight gain during this time, the recommendation for healthy-weight women is to aim for around 25-35 pounds for the duration of the pregnancy. These numbers vary slightly depending on whether you are carrying multiple babies, and whether you began your pregnancy over- or underweight. Most women gain between one and five pounds in the first trimester, and about a pound a week every week thereafter. After years of monitoring the scales and bemoaning additional weight, pregnancy is an enormously freeing time for many women. Enjoy this special time when every healthy choice you are making is benefitting your growing baby.

Fifteenth Week of Pregnancy

Now that you are fifteen weeks pregnant, the cat is probably out of the bag, and you can explain away all of your bizarre behaviors during the past few months. What can you expect from your baby and your body this week?

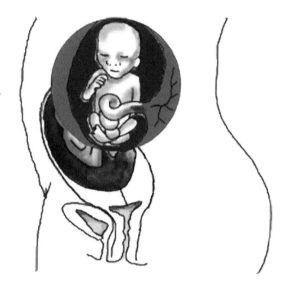

What is Going On with Your Baby at Fifteen Weeks Pregnant?

Baby is growing rapidly, and is now about the size of an apple--4 inches long from top to bottom, and weighing in around 2.5 ounces. Baby is drawing amniotic fluid in through the nose and into the upper respiratory sac, which fills the rudimentary air sacs that are present during lung development. Baby's legs are now longer than its arms, and can be moved at will along with all of the other joints and limbs. Eyelids may still be fused shut, but baby can sense light--moving away from a flashlight beamed at the belly is a very common response this week. Baby's taste buds are also forming and developing this week. If you were to schedule an ultrasound this week, the gender of your baby would likely be revealed, as all external sex organs are developed and distinct enough to be recognizable. However, most doctors will not schedule this particular ultrasound until between 18 and 20 weeks, so that the clarity of the picture is at its best and the results of its findings are more conclusive.

You may feel constantly as if your nose is stuffed up, or even be experiencing nosebleeds. These two conditions are very common during pregnancy and are jointly known as "rhinitis of pregnancy". Both are caused by hormonal changes resulting in increased vascularization and swelling of mucous membranes. This is a minor annoyance, to be sure, but an annoyance all the same.

You have probably gained a mere 5-7 pounds as of this week, which is pretty amazing, considering that you are nearly at the halfway point of your pregnancy.

Be sure to continue taking your prenatal vitamin. In addition to ensuring that your developing baby has everything it needs, the potent combination of prenatal vitamins and hormonal surges is probably having some side effects that non-pregnant women are sure to envy--namely, your suddenly lustrous and shiny hair, your glowing complexion, and your ability to grow your nails in record time.

Unfortunately, not ALL pregnant women reap these benefits- in fact some suffer from hormonal acne all throughout the course of pregnancy. When pregnant, you must be extra careful with how you treat this acne--some treatments, such as Accutane, are known to have harmful effects on a fetus and must not be used. Stick to the tried-and-true method of gentle cleansing, toning, and moisturizing, and invest in a good concealer for bad days. If you have decided to undergo an amniocentesis to further investigate any genetic concerns, sometime between now and 18 weeks is the time to schedule it. This procedure does come with some risk of miscarriage, so it is not usually performed unless absolutely vital; however, it can provide peace of mind regarding hundreds of genetic conditions and deformities.

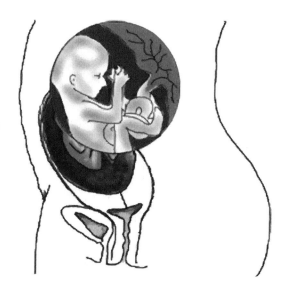

At sixteen weeks pregnant, you are four months along and rapidly approaching the halfway mark of your pregnancy. What can you expect this week?

What is Going On with Your Baby at Sixteen Weeks Pregnant?

Over the course of the next few weeks, your baby will undergo a rapid growth spurt, doubling its weight and adding inches to its crown-rump length. This week, baby is about 4.5 inches long from crown to rump, and weighs about 3.5 ounces--around the size of an avocado. Legs are more developed, eyes and ears are close to their final positions, and head is held almost erectly. Scalp patterning begins this week, though hair has yet to grow. Toenails are growing, and will continue through birth. Baby's heart is now pumping about 25 quarts of blood through his circulatory system; this amount will increase as development continues. Baby's ear bones are developed enough at this point that it is already able to hear and can distinguish its favorite sound of all--your voice--from other sounds.

Your uterus weighs nearly 9 ounces this week, and can be found about halfway between your pubic bone and your navel. Sixteen weeks is the earliest that you may begin to feel your baby's acrobatics.

This milestone, known as quickening, was once considered to be the first indication that the baby was showing signs of life. Those first few movements are enormously exciting for a pregnant woman, and belong to her alone, as they are not quite strong enough to be felt by anyone else. They have been compared to "gas bubbles," "butterflies in the tummy" or "popcorn popping".

Whatever metaphor comes to mind, these movements will be incredibly reassuring in the months to come, as they are an indication that your little one is alive and well. In later months, you will be performing a "kick count" in order to track your baby's state of health, but for now, simply enjoy the sensation of your little passenger making his or her presence felt.

At a doctor's appointment around this time, you will schedule the important ultrasound that will tell the doctor how your baby is developing, as well as the exciting news regarding your baby's gender. The best time for this appointment is around18-22 weeks--your OB/GYN will want to be sure that the picture is as clear as possible.

By 16 weeks, you may also notice an enlarging of veins in your legs due to increased blood volume and circulation. These prominent veins may likely turn into varicose veins, due to the increased pressure that your legs are under. Support hose may be helpful at this point, as will elevating your legs when possible and avoiding crossing them. Most varicose veins disappear shortly after delivery; those that linger can be taken care of with a variety of simple laser procedures.

During this week, you may also be offered an AFP (Alpha-Feto-protein) test, or "quad screen." This simple, non-invasive exam uses a sample of your blood sera to test for the presence of fetal proteins that may indicate a neural tube defect.

Seventeenth Week of Pregnancy

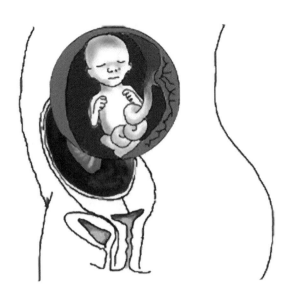

Now that you are seventeen weeks pregnant, you are beginning the second month of your second trimester. There is a lot to look forward to in the next few weeks, especially now that those pesky first-trimester symptoms are behind you.

What is Going On with Your Baby at Seventeen Weeks Pregnant?

This week, baby's skeleton is making the transition from carti-lage to bone, and the placenta is growing stronger and thicker. Baby weighs about 5 ounces and measures about 5 inches from crown to rump--around the size and weight of a red onion. Baby can freely move its joints, and sweat glands begin to develop. There is considerable movement in baby's aquatic home; you are probably feeling the effects of those tiny kicks and punches now, although they are still too weak to be felt by your partner at this point.

What is Going On with Your Body at Seventeen Weeks Pregnant?

As your abdomen enlarges due to the expanding uterus, your center of balance may begin to shift, increasing your likelihood of falling. In addition, pregnant women sometimes have a dif-ficult time adjusting to the parameters of their new bodies--be prepared to bang into just about everything from now until the end of your pregnancy and spend a significant amount of time laundering your shirts, as your enhanced cleavage and larger abdomen will be a magnet for spills of all kinds.

Continue to buckle up while in the car; despite the discomfort you may feel in restricting your belly, this is a vital safety measure that must be maintained. Buckle the belt tightly, and slip the shoulder portion over your belly to double up on the lap portion. During this time, try to be as careful as possible to protect your burgeoning belly. Wear low-heeled shoes with excellent traction, and limit your exercise to lower-impact activities.

Swimming and walking are two wonderful ways to maintain fitness while pregnant. At this point in your pregnancy, avoid all abdominal exercises that involve lying flat on your back. This is important, because at this stage, the weight of your uterus places pressure on blood vessels that deliver oxygen to the fetus. The plank position is a great one for pregnant women, and will strengthen your entire core, along with your shoulders and arms.

During the seventeenth week of pregnancy, you may notice your eyes becoming drier. The use of over-the-counter lubrication drops may alleviate this discomfort; if you wear contact lenses, switching to glasses for the remainder of your pregnancy may be the answer. By the end of this week, your baby will be developed enough for an ultrasound scan to be very accurate. If you are planning on learning the gender of your child, this could be the week to do it. Not all babies are cooperative in this respect--some maintain a modest crossed-leg position, making it impossible to distinguish the sex organs. Most OB/GYNs will not reschedule this ultrasound, as gender is not considered a vital statistic, but you may get lucky on the first try.

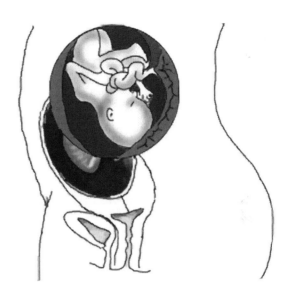

Now that you are eighteen weeks pregnant, there is no hiding your condition. You are probably well settled into your pregnancy, and excited about what is to come.

What is Going On with Your Baby at Eighteen Weeks Pregnant?

At 18 weeks, your baby weighs in at nearly half a pound, and is about 5.5 inches from crown to rump--approximately the size of a bell pepper. Baby is constantly moving around, and you are definitely feeling those kicks and punches by now. Baby's blood vessels are clearly visible through its thin skin. Its ears are perfectly situated now, and myelin is forming a protective covering around the nerves. By this week, baby girls have a fully formed uterus and Fallopian tubes, and baby boys have noticeable genitals. Baby can also yawn and hiccup now, important developments related to the central nervous system. In later weeks, you will be able to feel these hiccups as a series of rhythmic bumps low in your pelvis.

What is Going On with Your Body at Eighteen Weeks Pregnant?

By eighteen weeks, you are probably experiencing lower back pain due to the increased weight you are carrying in front of you. During pregnancy, try to seek natural homeopathic remedies for pain and colds. A hot bath may ease some of your discomfort, as may a cold pack or a hot rice pillow applied directly to the lower back.

During this time, a substance called relaxin is being released into your body to prepare you for the birth process. This relaxin makes your joints looser than when you are not pregnant, so do be careful when you are exercising not to overdo it. You may begin to notice stretch marks appearing on your breasts and belly; these can be extremely itchy. Stretch marks, unfortunately, are genetic, and if your mother had them, you are likely to have them as well. They will most likely fade once your baby arrives, but even if they do not, carry them with pride, as they are battle scars testifying that your amazing body has produced another life. Thick creams made with cocoa butter may temporarily aid with the itching.

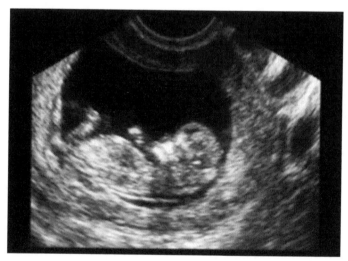
Ultrasound of a Fetus

Week 18 is probably the week you have been looking forward to--the week of your ultrasound. During this painless procedure, a variety of anatomical markers will be measured and recorded in order to check the progress of your baby.

The technician will cover your belly with a warm goo for better conductivity. She will then pass a wand over your belly, and the first picture of your precious baby will appear on the screen. She will measure your baby's femur length, which will help predict size and confirm due date. The level of your amniotic fluid will be measured, and the position and condition of the placenta will be noted. Now the fun part--the big reveal! Hopefully, baby will be cooperative, but he or she may be feeling shy, in which case changing position or prodding your belly may help uncross those little legs so you can get a peek at the sex organs. Most technicians will record portions of your session and put them on a DVD for you, as well as print out the very first snapshots of your sweet baby.

Nineteen weeks is a time of immense growth and development, both for you and for your baby. What is going on right now?

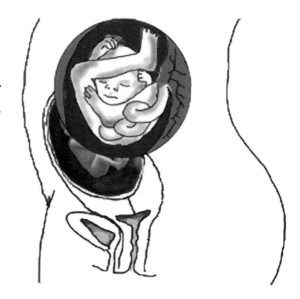

What is Going On with Your Baby at Nineteen Weeks Pregnant?

Baby's sensory development is progressing at a rapid rate. The brain is specializing areas for the five senses, and he or she is well able hear you. Some research suggests that a tune played repeatedly at this time will have soothing effects on the outside as your baby experiences recognition. This week, baby weighs a little over half a pound, and measures half a foot from top to bottom--about the size of a mango. Baby's body is covered with a waxy coating called the vernix caseosa, which protects its skin from the surrounding amniotic fluid. Arms and legs are in correct proportion to one another, and the first hair is growing on baby's head. This first hair will fall out soon after birth, and may grow back in an entirely different texture and color.

During this week, your body's swelling tissues are placing pressure on your nerves. You may experience sciatica, a radiating pain that follows your sciatic nerve in your lower back and radiates down to your upper thigh. Because your uterus is stretching to accommodate your baby's rapid growth, you may also experience a pain known as "round ligament pain." The round ligament supports the uterus, and when it stretches, it can feel like a sharp pain low in your abdomen. This is uncomfortable, but nothing to be concerned about unless it continues long after you have stopped moving; in a case like this, do contact your practitioner.

Skin changes are very common during this time, due to the extra estrogen in your system. The palms of your hands may be reddened, and you may notice a darkening of your nipples, freckles, underarms, and vulva, due to a temporary increase in pigmentation. When these darker patches appear on your cheeks and forehead, the condition is known as chloasma, or the "mask of pregnancy". It will disappear shortly after delivery, but in the meantime, protect your skin as much as possible with sunscreen and long sleeves. Most pregnant women, especially fair-skinned ones, notice a dark line running from right under the breastbone all the way down to the pubic bone. This is called the linea nigra, and will fade somewhat after delivery.

At your doctor's visit this month, you will listen to the heartbeat with the Doppler, the OB will measure your uterus from your fundus (top of the uterus) to track baby's growth, and your weight will be checked. At this point in your pregnancy, you should be up about 15 pounds.
Your urine will also be checked during each visit for the presence of proteins which indicate a possible urinary tract infection. These, as well as yeast infections, are quite common during pregnancy. In the instance of a UTI, there are many antibiotics that can be taken safely during pregnancy. Yeast infections can be treated with a variety of over-the-counter creams.

Drinking plenty of water can also aid in flushing your body of toxins and keeping these troublesome conditions at bay.

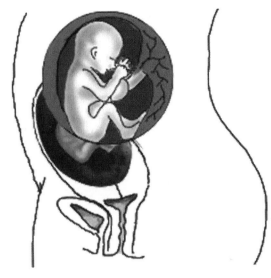

Twenty weeks is the halfway point of your pregnancy, as a full term pregnancy lasts around forty weeks. Less than 5% of women actually deliver on their due date, and the window of time for gestation is anywhere from 38 to 42 weeks; but for your sanity's sake, let us assume that we are at the halfway point. What can you expect in your twentieth week?

Twenty Weeks Pregnant- What is Going On with Your Baby?

Baby's measurements from this point on are taken from head to toe, as its legs are no longer curled up tightly against the torso. At 20 weeks, your baby is about 10 inches long from head to toe--about the length of a banana. Baby weighs in around 10.5 ounces, a little over half a pound. Baby is swallowing more and more amniotic fluid and developing his digestive system. Inside the bowels will be proof of these skills--a black, tarry substance called meconium that will show up in baby's first soiled diaper.

If you are having a boy, his testicles have started descending from the abdomen to their final position in the scrotum. Girls have a fully formed uterus, and around 7 million primitive eggs. Baby is practicing karate inside your belly regularly now, and those punches and kicks may be strong enough to be felt by your partner. Usually, baby's active times correspond with the times you are lying down, as your constant motion during the day is probably literally rocking him to sleep. These periods of alertness are in no way indicative of baby's life outside the womb, so do not be too concerned if your baby seems to be a night owl now.

Twenty Weeks Pregnant- What is Going On with Your Body?

Your uterus, now the size of a large cantaloupe, has left the pelvic cavity and is now expanding upward into the abdominal cavity, pushing aside your intestines and other organs. This is good news, as there is now less pressure on your bladder, and you may find that your trips to the bathroom are tapering off a bit. The fundus can be felt right at your belly button, and because of its positioning, your belly button may change from an innie to an outie.

It is a myth that the belly button only sticks out at the very end of pregnancy--in fact, most belly buttons are completely protruding around this time. If you dislike the look of your protruding navel, you may cover it with a bandage if you desire, but rest assured, it will back to normal shortly after delivery. Many women are hungrier than ever at this mid-point; try to keep your blood sugar stable with six small meals a day.

Keep drinking water, and make sure to get your daily walk or other exercise in. There are many workouts for pregnant women, including yoga and Pilates that are specially tailored to pregnancy. If you were not exercising before you discovered you were pregnant, do start gradually at this point--begin with daily walks, and slowly build to exercises of moderate intensity. Now is definitely not the time to be trying to lose weight or burn calories; you merely want to keep fit for the duration of your pregnancy.

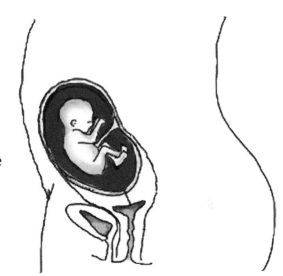

At twenty-one weeks, you are in the first week of the second half of your pregnancy, and time may seem to fly by as you continue to prepare for the biggest change you will ever experience in your life. What can you expect this week?

What is Going On with Your Baby at Twenty-One Weeks Pregnant?

Baby now weighs three-quarters of a pound, and is about 10.5 inches long--about the length of a sheet of paper. Its kicks and nudges are much stronger now; some of them may even be quite painful as baby uses your internal organs for target practice. Baby's eyebrows and eyelids are fully formed this week, and if you are having a girl, her vagina has begun to form, too. This week, baby's taste buds are beginning to develop, and he or she will likely be able to taste whatever you are eating. Go ahead and continue to eat the foods you enjoy--spicy, salty, or sweet; your baby will show its own tastes after it is born.

What is Going On with Your Body at Twenty-One Weeks Pregnant?

You may be up as much as 20 pounds at this point, and your body is definitely feeling it. Varicose veins may be appearing in your legs, and may run all the way up into your vulva. These bulgy, uncomfortable veins can be quite itchy and unsightly, but fear not--chances are they will be completely gone soon after delivery.

In the meantime, compression stockings may help, as will elevating your legs and keeping them uncrossed when at all possible. Another lovely side effect of pregnancy is constipation, which may lead to hemorrhoids if there is continued straining with bowel movements. Eat a diet high in fiber and whole grains, drink plenty of water, and if you are still uncomfortable, speak to your OB/GYN about a stool softener. At 21 weeks, because of the increased blood volume that comes with pregnancy, your blood pressure may be low. Be careful not to get up too quickly from a lying-down position, as you may feel dizzy or lightheaded. The best sleeping position for you at this point is lying on your left side, with a pillow nestled between your knees to properly align your back.

This week, the milk ducts in your breasts are producing colostrum--the first nutrition your baby will receive after the placenta is detached. Colostrum delivers concentrated nutrients to aid baby's small digestive system, and also contains a mild laxative to help your baby pass its first meconium stool.

Any time after twenty-one weeks, if your pregnancy has been deemed at high-risk for genetic defects, or if previous results from an amniocentesis were inconclusive, you may be offered a test known as "cordocentesis". This test is similar to an amniocentesis, but instead of sampling amniotic fluid, it samples fetal blood cells. There are some risks involved, so speak to your OB/GYN in order to weigh the risk factors with the benefits. The blood samples are tested for any chromosomal abnormalities, infections, or blood disorders and the results are usually available within 72 hours of the test.

Twenty-Second Week of Pregnancy

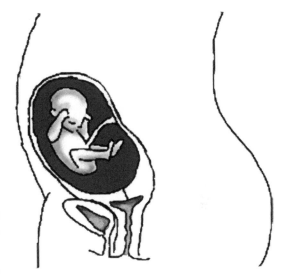

At twenty-two weeks, you are at the end of your fifth month, as hard as that is to believe. At this stage, when you are feeling relatively good, your pregnancy probably feels as if it is flying by too fast for you to get much done. Enjoy this sensation while it lasts; by the end of your pregnancy, each day will seem to take the entire nine months. What can you expect from your baby and your body this week?

What is Going On with Your Baby at Twenty-Two Weeks Pregnant?

Baby now looks like a miniature newborn, and is almost one pound in weight, and nearly a foot long. Tiny tooth buds are forming beneath the gums, although you will be able to enjoy a gummy smile for around 6 months before he or she cuts those teeth.

Lips, eyelids, and eyebrows are more and more distinct, although the color of the iris is yet to be determined. At birth, most Caucasian babies are blue-eyed, and most African-American, Asian, or Indian babies are brown-eyed. You must remember that eye color is a sex-linked gene, which means it is more variegated than other inherited traits. Your baby will attain his or her final eye color sometime around two years of age.

Baby's pancreas is now developing and beginning the production of some very important hormones. At 22 weeks, baby is covered with fine, downy hair called lanugo, and its skin is deeply wrinkled, awaiting the layers of fat that will form in later weeks.

What is Going On with Your Body at Twenty-Two Weeks Pregnant?

In addition to the ever-expanding belly, many pregnant women notice that their shoes are fitting snugly this week. This is partly due to the hormone relaxin, which causes ligaments to spread in preparation for delivery, including those in your feet, but it is also due to water retention and swelling, especially for those women who are reaching this stage in the summer months. Your shoe size may increase by as much as an entire size, and may not return to normal until after delivery.

This edema, or swelling, may also reach your fingers, so be sure to keep checking your rings; when they start to get uncomfortable, you may wish to remove them for safekeeping. Some women wear them on a chain around the neck, and others buy a replacement band in a larger size.

At twenty-two weeks, your round belly might be screaming at others for a rub--be prepared for your body to suddenly become public property.

If this makes you uncomfortable, you may back away, or simply ask others to keep their distance. If you have not found out the gender, be prepared for guesses from complete strangers based on how you are carrying, but rest assured, your shape has absolutely nothing to do with the gender of your child.

High or low, round or oblong, the way you carry is genetically predetermined and has nothing to do with baby's gender. The same goes for all of the other wives' tales such as the direction of a swinging wedding ring, whether your nose grows, or whether you crave sweet or salty. The only sure way to determine gender at this point is with an ultrasound or an amniocentesis.

Twenty-three weeks marks the beginning of your sixth month, meaning that you are almost at the end of your second trimester. There is a lot to look forward to in the next few weeks, but for now, enjoy where you are. What is going on with your baby and your body this week?

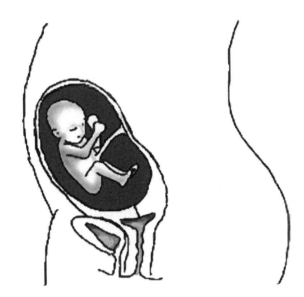

Twenty-Three Weeks pregnant- What is Going On with Your Baby?

By this week, baby's inner ear has developed enough to give him or her a sense of balance and positioning. When you sway to the music you hear, baby can feel you dance! Baby's acrobatics are very much evident now that he or she is so big; weighing a little over a pound and about a foot long, baby is now the approximate size of a large mango. Blood vessels inside baby's lungs are preparing for that first breath, and this week heralds the beginning of the time when baby really starts to pack on the pounds--by the end of this month, baby will have doubled its weight! By this week, any loud noises that occur frequently in your daily life will be old news for baby. This is good news, as it means that instead of terrifying him or her as a newborn, the vacuum cleaner may soothe him or her to sleep.

Twenty-Three Weeks Pregnant-
What is Going On with Your Body?

Did you forget your keys for the fifth time today? Blank out on someone's name? Leave the cupboard doors open without even realizing it? Go outside in your house slippers? You may have a case of "pregnancy brain". Caused by a rush of hormones, not to mention the baby who is the constantly growing source of your rapt attention, forgetfulness and absentmindedness are entirely normal during this time. Laugh it off, and realize that your brain will return to you once the baby has been born.

Other symptoms during this time are constant heartburn, swelling of the hands and feet, and erratic mood swings. Don't take antacids (especially Tums) to make the heartburn go away. Heartburn is a symptom that indicates poor digestion and the presence of acid reflux - taking the tablets only makes it worse. Taking antacids will reduce stomach acid and low stomach acid can lead to a leaky gut which causes other major issues.

Eating fermented foods, lifestyle changes eating 5 or 6 small meals a day, avoiding spicy or greasy food, and not lying down for 1 hour after eating will remedy the problem. Also eating yogurt and drinking milk.
Keep up the good work with your exercise routine, and as for mood swings, almost everyone in your life, from your boss to your spouse, will cut you extra slack during your pregnancy. If someone does make an insensitive comment, do try not to internalize it; you have more important things to be thinking about, like what color to paint the nursery. Take the high road, and try not to be stressed out.

Speaking of stress, this week would be a great week to begin putting into practice some serious relaxation techniques. Not only will this aid you in the short term to calm your busy mind, but it is also extremely important to have some inner reserves of peace stored for the big event of labor, especially if you choose to go with a natural birth. Even after the baby has been born, these techniques can help carry you through some tough adjustment periods and make your transition to motherhood that much happier. Yoga, meditation, and prayer are all excellent ways to tap into an inner serenity. Practice now, and when things start to get rough, you will be well prepared.

Twenty-Fourth Week of Pregnancy

Twenty-four weeks is an important week in the course of a pregnancy. For starters, this is the very first week in which your baby could potentially survive outside your body, if you were to have a preterm birth. Baby would need much specialized prenatal care, but there is a very good chance that he or she would be 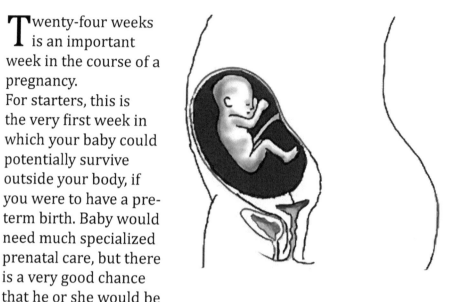 just fine in the long run. Before twenty-four weeks, there is virtually no chance of survival, and hospitals would not medically intervene, as this would be costly with very poor odds. What else is going on at twenty-four weeks?

What is Going On with Your Baby at Twenty-Four Weeks Pregnant?

Baby's growth is steady; he or she has gained nearly a quarter-pound in just one week, putting baby's total weight just over a pound, and total length at around a foot long. Baby has filled out some, but will pack on the pounds in the later weeks. Its brain is developing rapidly, and its taste buds are almost finished. Inside the lungs, "branches" are being formed on the respiratory "tree," as are cells that produce surfactant, which aid in inflation of the lungs. When you listen to your baby's heartbeat at your next appointment, it will be fast--about twice as fast as yours, measuring anywhere from 110 to 170 beats per minute.

Your weight gain is consistent at this point; you will be gaining around a pound a week. You may see numbers on the scale that you have never seen before, but this is not cause for alarm. You are growing a healthy baby, and most women lose their baby weight within a year of delivery, so focus on the positives, and try not to let the numbers scare you.

At twenty-four weeks, you will probably be screened for Gestational Diabetes. This simple test involves rapidly drinking a high-sugar content drink, (which tastes a bit like flat orange soda) and having blood drawn after an hour to measure how quickly the sugar is metabolized. If all goes well, you will be in the clear, but if you fail the first test, another one will be scheduled. This one will be a three-hour test, and you will have to fast before the test. If you fail this test as well, you will most likely be put on a restricted diet, and will have to test your blood each morning to maintain a safe blood sugar level. Gestational diabetes is a concern because it can lead to babies with low blood sugar and also may increase the probability of a Cesarean section, as it is a leading cause of macrosomia, or unusually large babies.

Your baby is nearly fully formed, but not ready to be born just yet. That is why, at this point, it is important to recognize the signs of preterm labor, which may be brought on by dehydration in some women. Be on the alert for more than five contractions in an hour, bright red spotting, swelling of the hands and feet, prolonged stomach pain, continuous vomiting, intense pelvic pressure, or your water breaking, and be sure to contact your OB/GYN immediately should any of these symptoms occur.

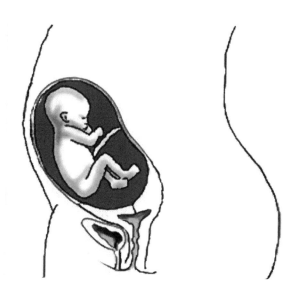

N ow that you are twenty-five weeks pregnant, you are well into your sixth month. What can you expect this week?

**What is Going On with Your Baby
at Twenty-Five Weeks Pregnant?**

Baby now weighs about a pound and a half and measures about 13.5 inches from head to toe. Baby is beginning to fill out more and more, and the next few weeks will see remarkable growth, as baby will more than quadruple his weight and add around 6 inches to his length. This week, baby's hair is growing more, and now has color and texture. Try not to get too attached to those dark curls, though--most babies lose nearly all of the hair that they are born with shortly after birth, and it may grow back in an entirely different color and texture. Under baby's skin and inside baby's lungs, capillaries are forming and filling with blood. Baby's nostrils, which until now have been plugged up, are now open, and his vocal cords are preparing for that first yell as he or she emerges into the world.

**What is Going On with Your Body
at Twenty-Five Weeks Pregnant?**

Due to a combination of factors, including slower digestion, constipation, and the weight of your uterus, you may still be suffering from hemorrhoids. These bulging veins in your rectum may be itchy, tender, and swollen, and are most definitely un-comfortable. Try sitting in a Sitz bath--a shallow pan filled with hot water. Applying witch hazel pads directly to the site, and per-haps affixing them to a panty liner, may also provide some relief. They will probably disappear soon after delivery—a sentence you are probably tired of hearing!

In addition to your regular exercise routine, it is important to strengthen your pelvic floor muscles in preparation for labor and delivery. These exercises, called Kegels, can be done anytime and anywhere. To perform a Kegel, tighten the muscles used to stop the flow of urine for ten seconds, squeezing the whole time. Release, and repeat. Try to work as many Kegels into your day as possible; do them in the shower, in front of the TV, even while sitting at a stoplight. The pelvic floor muscles act as a hammock, supporting the bladder, intestines, and uterus, and also main-tain continence as part of the urinary and anal sphincters. Pelvic floor muscles aid in the birthing process, as they cause the baby to rotate forward by providing resistance to the presenting part.

You may be feeling much heavier this week, as you are probably up around 20 pounds. Be kind to your feet during this time; save the spike heels, and instead choose low-heeled, supportive shoes or sneakers. Your back may also be plaguing you at this point. Ask your partner for a gentle massage, use a heated rice pillow for your lower back, and take frequent breaks during the day.

During your glucose screen last week, you may have had an iron count, which tests for anemia. Anemia can leave you feeling fatigued, the last thing you need at this point, so if your numbers came back low, be sure and ask your doctor to prescribe you some iron supplements.

Twenty-Sixth Week of Pregnancy

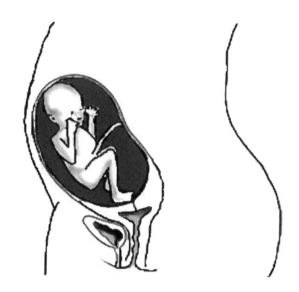

Twenty-six weeks is the last week of your sixth month, and the last week of your second trimester. Next week begins the last trimester in your amazing journey to mommyhood, and there are a lot of exciting changes to come. What can you expect this week?

What is Going On with Your Baby at Twenty-Six Weeks Pregnant?

The nerves inside baby's ear are more sensitive than ever. Not only can baby hear and respond to your voice, he or she is also starting to tune into dad's voice. If baby hears a loud noise, or a bright light is shined near your belly, baby's activity may noticeably increase. Baby's lungs are getting a workout this week, as he or she is practicing inhaling by taking in small amounts of amniotic fluid. Baby's growth spurt continues; he or she weighs about 2 2/3 pounds and measures about fourteen inches long. If baby is a boy, his testicles will descend into his scrotum in the next few days.

What is Going On with Your Body at Twenty-Six Weeks Pregnant?

This is the time to think about taking childbirth classes. Check the hospital where you will be delivering, as some offer a full slate of classes, and even labor and delivery room tours. It is not too early to write out a birth plan this week, but keep in mind that every birth is different, and the most important thing is to be flexible if circumstances do not play out according to your plan. At this point in your pregnancy, you are probably having a difficult time finding a comfortable sleeping position at night. This is especially true for habitual belly sleepers, as this is not a beneficial position for your body or your baby during this time. It is ideal to sleep on your left side, with a body pillow between your knees to maintain proper spinal alignment. You might find it helpful to prop up your breasts and/or your belly with another pillow for added support.

This week you may also notice an increase of leucorrhea, or vaginal discharge. Do not bother with scented wipes or douches, as they may irritate sensitive skin, but do wear a panty liner to maintain freshness.

This week or next you may start to experience Braxton Hicks contractions. These painless, short contractions occur when your brain sends a message to your body to prepare for labor. In response to these impulses, your uterus contracts. This may feel like tightening bands around your belly and last for several seconds. As your due date approaches, these "practice contractions" may become more intense, even painful. Practice your breathing, and try to change positions. If the contractions continue, or get closer together, and you find it difficult to talk through them, this may be preterm labor. Call your practitioner if you have any of the symptoms of preterm labor, such backache, pelvic pain, cramps, or your water breaking.

In addition to Braxton Hicks contractions, during this week you may be experiencing "restless leg syndrome," an uncontrollable twitching or tingling in the legs when you are lying down. Avoid caffeine, stretch your calf muscles, or sign up for a deep tissue massage from a certified prenatal masseur.

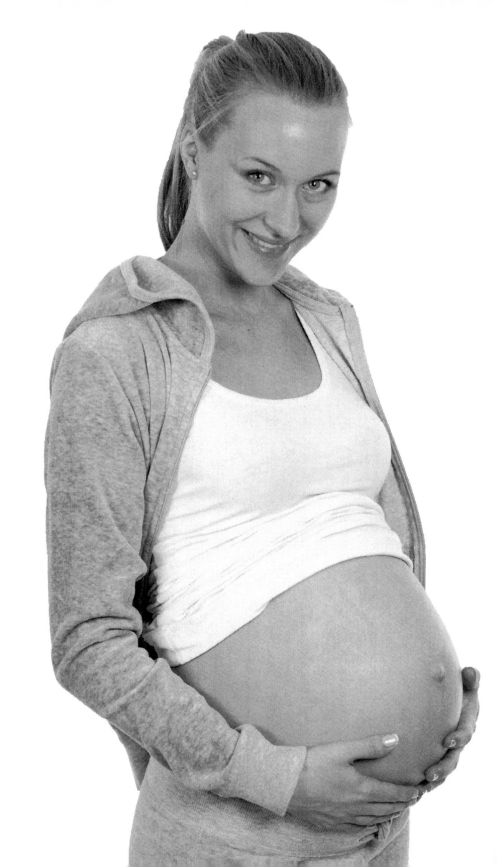

The Third Trimester

27 Week Pregnant – 40 Weeks Pregnant

The Third Trimester is the period during which you must prepare to give birth to your child. You may be feeling heavy and fed-up with pregnancy, especially throughout these final three months. It is likely that you also feel somewhat anxious about the birthing process.

Keep reading to discover what is going on inside your body week by week:

Twenty-Seven weeks is the first week of month seven, and the beginning of your third trimester. By now, the harsh reality of your impending labor may be hitting home, or you may still be riding high from the relatively easy second trimester. Either way, take a look at what you can expect this week?

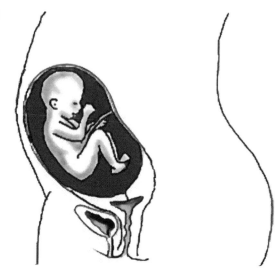

Twenty-Seven Weeks Pregnant- What is Going On with YourBaby?

At twenty-seven weeks, baby weighs about the same as a head of cauliflower--nearly two pounds. He or she is about 14.5 inches from head to heels. Baby's brain is very active this week, as more and more brain tissue develops. Lung development is nearly complete, and every week that passes from this point on indicates a greater chance of survival were your baby to be born early. Baby has periods of activity interspersed with quiet periods, and can suck its fingers and open and close its eyes. You may be able to feel baby's hiccups--tiny, rhythmic bumps deep in your lower abdomen.

Twenty-Seven Weeks Pregnant- What is Going On with Your Body?

As you segue into the third trimester, you will carry over many of the symptoms of the first two trimesters, including heartburn, constipation, frequent urination, insomnia, and restlessness at night.

However, you are probably enjoying some things about pregnancy this week, such as your long, shiny hair, your fast-growing fingernails, and your glowing complexion. All of these "pregnancy perks" are slight compensation for the other not-so-pleasant symptoms of pregnancy, so enjoy them while they last!

At this point in the pregnancy, you are probably up around 20-25 pounds. For those who have always been body-conscious, seeing those numbers on the scale can be a scary thing. Now is not the time to diet or over-exert yourself in an attempt to control your weight gain--if you have been eating sensibly and maintaining your exercise regime, the weight will come off with few problems soon after you deliver your baby.

In the meantime, focus on where that weight is going and what it is being used for- you are creating a whole new life inside you! Baby is extremely active now, and is running out of room, which means that those acrobatics may pack quite a punch. Baby also might find one particular spot, such as your bladder, and kick at it repeatedly. Enjoy this time; as strange as it may sound, many women report a feeling of hollowness once the baby has been born— to have another life growing inside of you is a sensation like no other.
This week, continue practicing your calming skills in preparation for the not-so-calm events yet to come. Write up your birth plan, and bring it to your next doctor's appointment so that your practitioner can look over it.

This week is also a great time to start thinking about planning your maternity leave, if you are employed. Sit down with an HR representative as soon as possible, and figure out the best plan for you. Some women go back about 8 weeks after delivery, others terminate their employment for the 24/7 job of motherhood; however you decide to do it, it is best to plan your leave in advance.

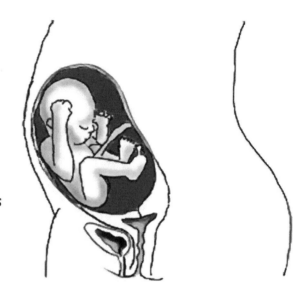

At twenty-eight weeks pregnant, you are closer than ever to your delivery date. A baby born this week has a 90% chance of survival, but would obviously fare much better the longer he or she stays inside. What can you expect this week?

What is Going On with Your Baby at Twenty-Eight Weeks Pregnant?

At twenty-eight weeks, your baby is probably settling into its final, head-down position. There is very little room for your not-so-little little one now, so chances are, once it is head-down it will stay that way. Do not despair if your baby is still in a breech position by this week; there is still time for it to flip, and if not, there are certain measures your doctor can take to increase your chances of a vaginal birth. Baby weighs around 2.5 pounds, and is almost 16 inches long--4 inches shy of being finished! Baby has eyelashes now, and can blink, cough, suck, hiccup, and take breaths. When baby sleeps, it now has an REM (rapid eye movement) phase just like you, which means he or she may already be dreaming!

What is Going On with Your Body at Twenty-Eight Weeks Pregnant?

You will be visiting your OB/GYN more frequently now, about

every two weeks instead of every four. He or she will continue to monitor your blood pressure, listen to the baby's heartbeat, record your weight gain, measure your fundal height, and check for protein in your urine. If protein is discovered in your urine at this point and you additionally have an elevated blood pressure reading, you may be diagnosed with preeclampsia.

Preeclampsia is a condition that affects between three and eight percent of pregnant women and causes blood vessels to constrict and deliver less blood to vital organs such as the liver, kidneys, and brain. When less blood flows to your uterus, it causes problems with the baby, stunting its growth, and leaving it with too little amniotic fluid. This can even cause placental abruption (the placenta detaching from the uterine wall before delivery).

The only cure for preeclampsia is immediate delivery of the baby. Fortunately for the majority of women, the condition shows up much later in pregnancy. Signs to watch for are swelling in the face or hands, called edema, sudden weight gain (more than four pounds in a week), headaches, dizziness, nausea, or extreme pain in your upper abdomen. Should any of these symptoms occur, contact your practitioner immediately.

The top of your uterus can now be felt around three inches above your navel, and you are probably feeling extremely heavy and large. Wondering how much bigger you can get? The next few weeks will be a time of rapid growth for you and you baby; as the little one packs on the weight, so will you. Expect to gain around two pounds a week from here on out. Facing downward in your pelvis, baby's head may be putting pressure on your sciatic nerve. This nerve runs from your lower back all the way down your thigh. It can be excruciating to experience sciatic nerve pain, or sciatica, so try to shift position and hope that baby does the same.

Twenty-Ninth Week of Pregnancy

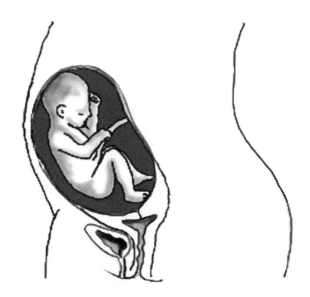

What is Going On with Your Baby at Twenty-Nine Weeks Pregnant?

At twenty-nine weeks, baby now tips the (imaginary) scales at 2.5 pounds--about the same weight as a butternut squash. From head to toe, it measures just over 15 inches long. This week, more development goes into the muscles and lungs, and the head is slowly increasing in size to make room for that burgeoning brain. Because baby is big by now, its movements will be more pronounced beneath the surface of your belly. You may be able to discern actual body parts--a rounded bottom, a sharp knee or elbow, or the bulge of baby's back. Baby's increasing nutritional needs dictate that you should increase your intake of protein, vitamin C, folic acid, and iron. Calcium is also important during this time, as baby's little bones are soaking it up. As with every nutrient and especially calcium, your baby will take what he needs from YOU--meaning that if there is a shortage of some essential nutrient, you will be the one who feels it, not the baby.

Welcome to the self-sacrificial world of motherhood--and remember to drink that milk!

What is Going On with Your Body at Twenty-Nine Weeks Pregnant?

You may have gained up to 25 pounds by now, and the weight is definitely taking its toll on you. An aching back, swollen feet, and slow gait are all common for pregnant women at this stage. You may also experience dizziness and light-headedness when you get up too suddenly, so do take your time. In order to rise from a fully prone position, it will be necessary to "log roll" onto your side to get up--no more sit ups for you at this stage of the game! Many pregnant women opt to get regular pedicures during the third trimester; reaching your feet is nearly impossible by now, yet having perfectly painted toenails seems to be high on the priority list when thinking about going into labor.

While you may feel massive and unattractive, chances are your partner is anything but turned off by you. Most men find the sight of a pregnant woman, especially THEIR pregnant woman, extremely sexy, as it affirms their own virility and masculinity. While sexual relations can be very satisfying at this point in pregnancy, and indeed may help with some of your symptoms, extra communication is required to make the experience pleasurable for both. This late in the pregnancy, you should not be on your back for more than a few minutes, as you may experience shortness of breath and the weight of your uterus will threaten the baby's blood supply. In addition, air must not be introduced into the vagina, due to the risk of an embolism. Furthermore, your breasts may be tender and sore still; although your partner may wish to caress them, this may be a decided turn-off for you. Positions in which both partners are on their sides should be the easiest way in which to continue your lovemaking sessions all the way until your due date, should it be mutually desired.

Now that you are thirty weeks pregnant, you have passed a significant milestone. The end of your pregnancy is just a few short weeks away! You are nearly into your eighth month, and are probably wondering what is in store for you this week.

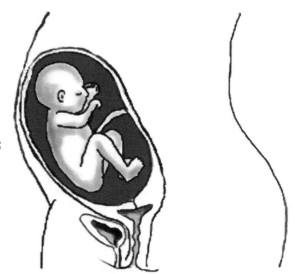

What is Going On with Your Baby at Thirty Weeks Pregnant?

Baby weighs nearly three pounds now, about the size of a head of cabbage, and is nearly 16 inches long. About 1.5 pints of amniotic fluid surround your baby, although this volume will decrease significantly in the coming weeks as baby gets bigger and takes up more space. Eyesight is developing, and baby can respond to light, even though at birth it will only be able to see about 8 inches in front of it (the approximate distance from your breasts to your face). Weight gain is increasing, as baby continues gaining about half a pound a week, and the grooves in the brain are nearly fully formed. Baby is able to regulate his body temperature now, so the lanugo (the fine, downy hair that covers his body) is starting to disappear.

Your constant companion these days is heartburn, which has definitely kicked up a notch since the early days. As your body prepares to deliver your baby, the muscles in your pelvis start to spread, due to the influence of the hormone relaxin. This hormone also influences other muscles, such as the muscle that separates the stomach from the esophagus. Because this muscle is more relaxed, stomach acid can reenter the esophagus, making your days uncomfortable, and your nights nearly unbearable. Ask your OB/GYN for an indigestion prescription a bit stronger than the over-the-counter tablets you may have been relying on up to this point.

At thirty weeks, you may wish to start researching the possibility of cord-blood banking or donation. Why is cord blood so important? Cord blood contains stem cells which have yet to be differentiated, so that they can be manipulated in a laboratory setting to assume the functionality of wherever they are placed, thus creating enormous potential to treat certain diseases. The cord blood is what is left in the placenta and umbilical cord after the birth of your baby. If you decide to donate or bank it, it will be collected painlessly after the birth of your baby. There are many private companies that will store it for you, should you decide to bank it for your family's own use. If you decide to donate, all that is required is a consent form. Your baby could give another child the gift of life, just by virtue of being born.

Your second trimester stamina has probably long vanished, as you are most likely struggling with both fatigue and insomnia. Do not be afraid to ask for help during this time, and take frequent breaks during the day whenever you can. Your uterus is about four inches above your navel, and your weight is probably up around 30 pounds by this point. Weight gain should be fairly consistent over the next few weeks, with a slow-down or even reversal as the big day approaches.

Thirty-First Week of Pregnancy

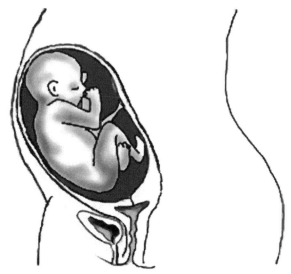

Throughout a pregnancy, a woman experiences many changes, both physically and emotionally. Hormonal changes may seem more pronounced during the early stages, tapering off by 20 or 30 weeks. At thirty-one weeks pregnant, most moms-to-be are becoming a little anxious for Junior to arrive. These final weeks of pregnancy can be uncomfortable and a bit tense, especially if this is your first pregnancy.

What is Going On with Your Baby at Thirty-One Weeks Pregnant?

After thirty-one weeks of pregnancy, the developing baby may gain up to eight ounces per day until reaching full term. The average baby will weigh about three pounds as the mom reaches thirty-one weeks of pregnancy. As the womb is limited to accommodate the growing baby, he or she will be drawn into the fetal position at about 30 or 31 weeks. Although baby's brain, heart, and other organs are nearly mature, its lungs have not developed enough to function at full capacity outside of the womb. At 31 weeks pregnant, the mom-to-be can expect her bun in the oven to require a little more preparation.

At thirty-one weeks pregnant, the mom-to-be may begin to feel slightly more sensitive to certain foods or scents. Heartburn, nausea, and upset stomach are not uncommon at 31 weeks pregnant. Certain foods that have never caused issues before the pregnancy may begin to cause stomach distress. A good way to deal with these minor issues is to cut back on sodium, as well as fatty or fried foods. If spicy or acidic foods are causing upset stomach or acid indigestion, it may be best to avoid them as well. It is also a good idea to eat frequent mini meals during the last few months of pregnancy, rather than three full-sized meals a day.

Most pregnant women have heard of Braxton Hicks contractions. These are basically mild contractions which can be felt midway through a pregnancy. By thirty-one weeks, Braxton Hicks uterine contractions may occur more frequently, although they are not usually a sign that labor is imminent. However, whenever uterine contractions occur more than three times per hour, it is best to contact a physician or medical care provider.

When mild Braxton Hicks contractions occur infrequently at thirty-one weeks, there are simple measures that may ease the discomfort. A warm water bottle placed on the tummy may help relax uterine muscles. Additionally, a warm bath may also induce relaxation, especially before bedtime. Some women find that taking a short walk may also dispel the sensations of Braxton Hicks contractions. Under a physician's recommendation, some light stretching exercises may additionally be helpful.

It is inevitable that at thirty-one weeks pregnant the mom to be will experience her fair share of aches and pains at the end of the day. The baby will begin to be more active, often shifting its little body or kicking up a storm. As for mom, lower back pain is not uncommon in the thirty-first week of pregnancy, and achy, tired legs are also to be expected. Take heart; there are only nine more

weeks of aches and bloating before that precious bundle of joy makes his or her grand debut.

Thirty-Second Week of Pregnancy

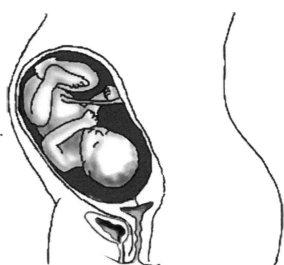

Now that you are thirty-two weeks pregnant, you are definitely in the home stretch. You have only eight weeks left in your pregnancy, and time seems as though it has flown. What can you expect this week of your pregnancy?

What is Going On with Your Baby at Thirty-Two Weeks Pregnant?

This week, baby weighs about a quarter-pound shy of four pounds--about the size of a jicama. Head to toe, baby measures a little over 16.5 inches long- meaning that there is not a whole lot of wiggle room left for him or her. Baby has now entered the weight gaining phase, and will gain a third to a half of his birth weight over the next 7 weeks, most of it in the form of fat deposits under the skin. Baby has toenails, fingernails, and hair on its head and its skin is losing that wrinkled look as fat accumulates. The downy lanugo is being shed, and baby is nearly ready to be born. A baby born this week would have an excellent chance of survival outside the womb.

What is Going On with Your Body at Thirty-Two Weeks Pregnant?

To meet your body's and your baby's growing demands, your blood volume has increased up to 50 percent since the beginning of your pregnancy. Your uterus, now about five inches above your belly button, is pushing up on your diaphragm and crowding your stomach and other internal organs. The consequence of this is shortness of breath and even more heartburn. Try sleeping propped up on pillows to relieve some of your discomfort. If you are still exercising this far along, take it easy. The purpose of exercise at this point is to maintain flexibility and relieve stress, not to lose weight, so do not overexert yourself at this stage. Continue gentle stretching and strengthening exercises, as well as performing Kegels to strengthen the pelvic floor in preparation for labor and delivery.

Because of your increasing weight and changing center of gravity, you may be suffering from constant back pain these days. If the pain comes on suddenly and radiates around to the front of your abdomen in the form of cramping, it may be a sign of pre-term labor. Be sure to call your OB/GYN should you have any lower back pain that turns into cramping. Spotting at this point should be mentioned to your practitioner, as well.

One common complaint of pregnant women at this point is itchy skin on the abdomen. About one in two hundred women develop a hive-like rash called PUPPS (pruritic urticarial papules and plaques). This common pregnancy dermatitis has no lasting effect on mom or baby, but is annoying due to its extreme itchiness. The papules usually begin on the abdomen, many times within existing stretch marks, and then spread to the legs, arms, and neck. Interestingly enough, nearly 70% of women who suffer from PUPPS deliver boys. The condition is usually treated with water-based emollient lotions such as Vaseline or Aquaphor, and in severe cases, with topical or oral corticosteroids.

Thirty-Third Week of Pregnancy

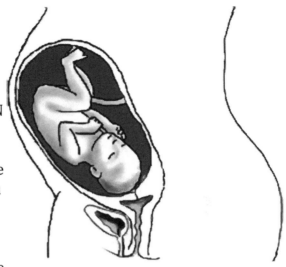

Now that you are in your thirty-third week, you have begun your eighth month of pregnancy. You should be seeing your OB/GYN every week by now, hearing your sweet baby's heartbeat on the Doppler each time. You have probably gained nearly 30 pounds by now, and are wondering what else is in store for you this week.

What is Going On with Your Baby at Thirty-Three Weeks Pregnant?

This week, baby tips the scales at around 4 pounds (about the weight of a pineapple), and is a little bit longer than 17 inches from head to heel. Baby's skeleton is hardening, although the bones in its skull are not yet fused together, which allows the pieces to overlap so baby's skull can fit more easily through the birth canal. You will be very grateful for this fact in just a few weeks! The skull bones will fuse in early adulthood, after the brain and other tissues have reached their final size. Baby is so big at this point that the level of amniotic fluid has reached its highest point. This means that baby's acrobatics and attempts to "bend it like Beckham" can be felt much more intensely, as there is less fluid to cushion the blows. This week, antibodies are being passed from you to baby to beef up baby's immune system in preparation for his exit into the germy world that we call home.

What is Going On with Your Body
at Thirty-Three Weeks Pregnant?

This week heartburn and shortness of breath are still going strong. You are almost at the finish line. Hang on...you are nearly there! Don't take antacids especially Tums. Heartburn is a symptom that indicates poor digestion and the presence of acid reflux - taking the tablets only makes it worse. Taking antacids will reduce stomach acid and low stomach acid can lead to a leaky gut which causes other major issues. Eating fermented foods, lifestyle changes eating 5 or 6 small meals a day, avoiding spicy or greasy food, and not lying down for 1 hour after eating will remedy the problem. Also eating yogurt and drinking milk.

Some women have the misfortune to have a recurrence of morning sickness during the third trimester; this will be less intense than in the first trimester, but still unpleasant. Follow the guidelines that helped you get through the early weeks, such as eating small meals more frequently, sucking on ginger candy, and upping your water intake to avoid dehydration.
Insomnia is also common in these last few weeks; the combination of frequent urination, achy back, indigestion, and increased fetal activity at night all conspire to beat the Sandman around this time. If possible, try to nap during the day, and avoid caffeine after your morning cup of coffee, as caffeine exacerbates insomnia.

Right around now, you may be asked to perform a kick count on your baby. This simply means that you count how many kicks, punches, and rolls that your little acrobat performs in the space of an hour. This test lets your OB/GYN know that everything is all right in there. If the number is less than 10, drink a glass of orange juice and perform the count again. If your kick count comes up low several times, you may be asked to come in for an assessment, including a non-stress test (NST), and maybe even a third trimester ultrasound. A baby born at thirty-three weeks has an extremely good chance of being entirely healthy, so you may even be scheduled for an induction if conditions inside your womb are deteriorating.

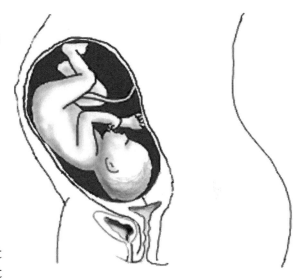

Now that you are thirty-four weeks pregnant, you are in full-fledged waddling mode. You are probably thoroughly sick of your tried-and-true maternity wear, and wondering if you will ever be back to your normal self. Fear not! In just about six short weeks, you will forget all of these cares as you gaze into your perfect newborn's beautiful eyes for the first time. What is in store for your baby and your body this week?

What is Going On with Your Baby at Thirty-Four Weeks Pregnant?

Baby now weighs a few ounces under five pounds (think of the weight of a bag of flour), and measures a good 18 inches from head to heel. Fat layers are smoothing out your baby's skin, which will aid in temperature regulation outside the womb. Baby's central nervous system and lungs are maturing, and the vernix (the cheesy coating that protects baby's skin from his surrounding watery environment) is at its thickest. Fingernails are fully formed, and will probably be ready to trim after baby is delivered. Babies born between now and thirty-seven weeks have just as much of a chance to survive and thrive as those born at full term (thirty-nine weeks). If born now, baby might require a short stay in the neonatal unit, but most probably will not suffer any long-term disadvantages due to prematurity.

What is Going On with Your Baby at Thirty-Four Weeks Pregnant?

Your back hurts, your stretch marks are itchy, and people have probably begun asking you when that baby will ever be born. These last few weeks can be incredibly taxing for a pregnant woman, especially a first-timer, when fears about labor and delivery cluster at the forefront of the mind. If you have not yet signed up for a class at your birthing center, doing so may help ease some of your anxieties as you learn the stages of labor, and what to expect the day you arrive at the hospital. Educating yourself through reading may help, as may speaking with people in your life who have already given birth. Hold fast to the knowledge that women have been having babies for millennia, and in far worse conditions than you will find yourself when the big day finally arrives. Believe in your own strength and the strength of your body to deliver your baby safely.

This late in your pregnancy, you will most likely be seeing your practitioner once a week. Your weight gain should be holding steady at about a pound a week (more than half of that will go directly to the baby). Your uterus will be measured during these appointments, and should be felt five to six inches above the navel. It is perfectly common to be measure somewhat higher or lower; if the discrepancy is exceptional, a third-trimester ultrasound may be scheduled in order to more closely gauge the baby's due date.

This week, in preparation for your baby's arrival, make sure you have a car seat and know how to install it. Your local police or fire station can install it for you the first time, so you know the proper method.

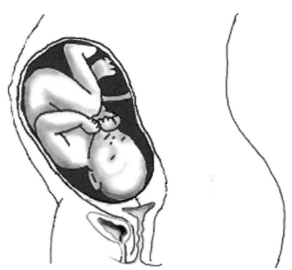

At thirty-five weeks pregnant, you are on the very last week before your last month of pregnancy. Baby could arrive at any time now, and many women choose to begin their maternity leave this week, in order to prepare for imminent labor without the stress that working full-time can add. What is in store for your baby and your body this week?

What is Going On with Your Baby at Thirty-Five Weeks Pregnant?

There is not much room left in your womb now, as at this point there is more baby than amniotic fluid. Baby is over 18 inches long from head to heels, and weighs in at a little over five pounds. Baby's movements will change from rolling and somersaulting to kicks and punches at this point, as there is no longer enough space for acrobatics. This is a good thing, as hopefully baby is in the head-down position at this point, and is likely to remain so in preparation for birth. Kidneys are fully developed, lungs are nearly mature, and baby's liver is able to process waste products. The next few weeks will see mostly the addition of fat stores, as your baby is nearly developmentally complete.

What is Going On with Your Body at Thirty-Five Weeks Pregnant?

Expect vision changes this week, as hormones released during pregnancy can cause dry eyes, and even change the shape of your eye lens, rendering you temporarily near- or far-sighted. No need to be alarmed; these changes will disappear after the birth of your baby, which is looming closer and closer. Sometime between now and thirty-seven weeks, a Group B Strep test will be performed at your weekly doctor's appointment. This simple test checks for the presence of Group B Streptococcus bacteria, which colonize the rectum and vaginal canal of some women. Though not harmful to a pregnant woman, a baby passing through a birth canal where these bacteria are present may experience complications such as pneumonia. If bacteria are found, an intravenous antibiotic will be administered to you during the birth of your baby, to ensure that he or she remains bacteria-free.

This week, in preparation for labor, you might ask your partner to begin perineal massage on you. This simple technique prepares the body for labor, and may help prevent painful tears and lacerations during the birthing process. To perform a perineal massage, have your partner thoroughly wash his hands. Then, have him warm a little olive oil or lubricant in his hands, and gently massage your perineum by placing his thumbs about an inch inside your vagina, pressing downward and to the sides at the same time. Have him continue this gentle stretching for about two minutes. Performed twice a day for the last few weeks of pregnancy, this massage technique has been proven to increase perineal flexibility and reduce the need for an episiotomy.

Because the arrival of a new baby is an extremely stressful and busy time, these last few weeks of pregnancy are an excellent time for you to make and freeze meals, pre-address and stamp announcement envelopes, and wash and fold all of baby's teeny-tiny onesies.

Thirty-Sixth Week of Pregnancy

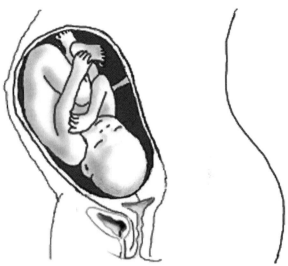

Now that you are in your thirty-sixth week of pregnancy, you are officially in your final month. At the end of this week, you will be technically full-term, as "full-term" is a time frame that ranges from thirty-seven to forty-two weeks. Your baby may arrive at any time during that window. A baby born at thirty-six weeks would have absolutely no long-term troubles, and only a small chance of being admitted to the NICU for a short time. What can you expect from your baby and your body this week?

What is Going On with Your Baby at Thirty-Six Weeks pregnant?

Baby is still rapidly gaining weight at the rate of about an ounce a day. He or she now tips the scales at around six pounds, and is more than 18.5 inches from head to heel. The downy covering of hair is being shed this week, as is most of the vernix caseosa. Both of these, as well as other secretions, are swallowed by your baby along with amniotic fluid, and will re-appear as meconium, your baby's first bowel movement. Your baby should already be in a head-down position in preparation for birth, but if he or she is being stubborn about it, your practitioner may suggest scheduling an "external cephalic version," which is a form of manipulating the baby's position externally, in hopes of turning the baby around.

Since baby is so large at this point, your internal organs, including your stomach, have been pushed aside to accommodate your uterus. This means that you may find it difficult to eat a normal-sized meal. During this time, smaller meals should be the rule-of-thumb for you.

This week, baby may start to descend into your pelvis, or "drop." This is great news, as heartburn may significantly decrease and feelings of breathlessness may subside now that baby is situated lower. The bad news is, once baby drops, you will probably feel increased pressure in your lower abdomen, meaning that you will need to urinate more frequently and have to waddle around, as increased vaginal pressure makes you feel as if you are carrying a bowling ball between your legs.

You may notice that your Braxton Hicks contractions are more frequent now. This late in pregnancy, what you believe to be Braxton Hicks may instead be full-on contractions, signifying that labor has begun. Remember that Braxton Hicks contractions, even if they are strong and uncomfortable, will usually subside if you change position (from lying down to standing, for example). True labor contractions will continue despite all efforts. Be sure to review the early signs of labor with your practitioner and know when to contact him or her. As a general rule, call the doctor if your contractions follow a 1, 5, 1 pattern—that is, one minute long contractions, with five minutes in between, for one hour.

This late in your pregnancy, it is unadvisable (not to mention extremely uncomfortable) to venture farther than your hometown. Most airlines will not let a woman fly when she is in her final month, for fear of an in-flight "spectacle" that is entirely unplanned, so stick close to home and prepare for your little one's imminent arrival.

Thirty-Seventh Week of Pregnancy

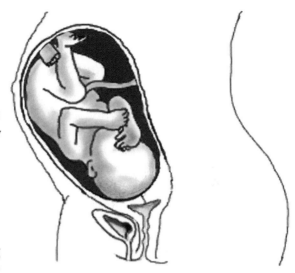

Now that you are thirty-seven weeks pregnant, you are officially considered full-term. Congratulations! This means that your baby could arrive any time between now and forty-two weeks. You may be chomping at the bit to give birth, or you may be feeling frantic at the thought of all you have left to accomplish, but either way, the end is near, and you will be holding your precious newborn in your arms very soon.

What is Going On with Your Baby at Thirty-Seven Weeks Pregnant?

Since baby is now considered full-term, its lungs will, in all probability, be mature enough to adjust to life outside your womb. Some babies may not be quite ready, so if you are scheduling a C-section, it should not be for another two weeks unless medically necessary. This week, baby weighs in at a little over six pounds, and measures a little over 19 inches. Baby now has a full head of hair, anywhere from half an inch to 1.5 inches long.

What is Going On with Your Body at Thirty-Seven Weeks Pregnant?

At this week's appointment, and all the rest of your appointments from now until the big day, your practitioner will be looking for signs of labor. He or she will take note of your baby's position in relation to the pelvis, known as engagement, and whether effacement, or thinning, of your cervix has begun. The practitioner may perform a fingertip check to see whether your cervix is dilated at all. Each of these factors is assigned a value, and together, they give your practitioner a relatively good idea of when labor will begin. There are no guarantees, however. Baby has his or her own special timing, and you may be stuck at a certain stage of dilation or effacement for hours, days, or weeks.

You should review the signs of labor with your practitioner, and have an overnight bag ready for your hospital stay from this point on. One sign that labor is nearing is the loss of your mucous plug.

This slimy pink tissue has served as a physical barrier protecting the womb from bacteria and other threats. Once the cervix starts thinning and opening, it may fall out.

Another sign that labor is imminent is the breaking of your water. You may have seen movies in which a pregnant woman's water breaks, and she instantly starts screaming as she goes into labor. Chances are, that will not be your story, as fewer than 15% of women experience the rupture of their membranes before the onset of labor. Even if your water does break, contractions may not start immediately. In either case, notify your practitioner. If your contractions have not begun twenty-four hours after your water has broken, you will be induced early to prevent infection in the baby.

It may be a good idea at this point to select a family member or close friend and make sure that they have keys to your place, as well as a list of contact information. This individual can be the point person while you are in the hospital, and get the phone chain started when you go into labor.

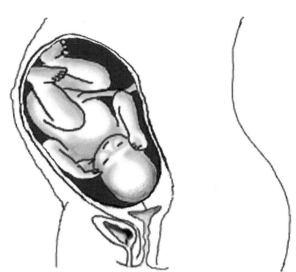

When you are thirty-eight weeks pregnant, time seems to stand still. Two weeks feels like a lifetime away as you nervously await the onset of labor. What else can you expect this week?

What is Going On With Your Baby at Thirty-Eight Weeks Pregnant?

At nearly seven pounds and 19.5 inches from head to heel, baby is close to his or her final weight and length. Baby now has the ability to grasp at objects, meaning that he or she will be able to clutch your finger immediately after birth, making your heart swell with motherly pride. All of baby's systems are up and running, waiting for the signal to launch, which could come any day now. Final touches are still taking place during the final weeks of gestation, such as shedding of the lanugo and vernix, fine-tuning the nervous system in preparation for the coming influx of outside stimuli, producing more surfactant in the lungs in preparation for the first breath, and gaining yet more fat. For all intents and purposes, your baby is fully "cooked," and waiting for the hormonal signal that will send it on its way.

You are exhausted, sick and tired of waddling around like a penguin, and you just may have to stab the next person who tells you that you look ready to pop. Welcome to the end of your pregnancy! The fear of impending labor may render you sleepless with anxiety, so now is the time to practice your calming and centering. Whenever you feel the panic begin to set in, remind yourself that you are strong, your doctors are capable, and your body knows what it is doing. Women have been birthing babies since the beginning of time, and you WILL be fine.

Keep your bag packed and ready for your hospital trip, as it could come at any time, and the last thing you will want to do between contractions is spend time locating your lucky socks.

Some things that may be useful to have during labor and recovery are: ChapStick, hard candy, cozy socks, your iPod (with a "birthing mix" of upbeat, soothing, or favorite tunes), a tennis ball (extremely useful for lower back massage in the event of back labor), baby's going-home outfit (choose newborn size, as 0-3 months will most likely be too big), going-home clothes for you (your best bet are the maternity clothes you wore at six months pregnant), a nursing bra or cami, and toiletries and makeup for those first family snapshots.

Be sure that your car seat is installed by this week of your pregnancy, as this is one less to worry about as the big day looms closer. All cars manufactured after September 1, 2002, have what is known as the LATCH system (Lower Anchors and Tethers for Children), making car seat installation fairly simple. If you have any problems, head over to your local fire or police department, and someone will install it for you—your hard-earned tax dollars are put to work at last!

N ow that you are thirty-nine weeks pregnant, your due date is fast approaching. You are in the home stretch now, and probably wondering if this pregnancy is EVER going to end. Remember, only 15% of pregnant women actually deliver on their due dates; this 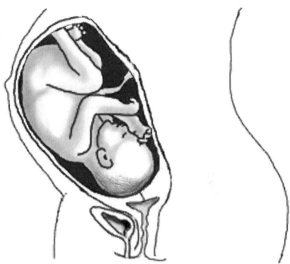 could mean that your baby is content to be inside you and will stay until an eviction notice is posted in the form of an induction. What can you expect this week?

What is Going On with Your Baby at Thirty-Nine Weeks Pregnant?

Not much is happening this week, as baby is fully formed, functional, and simply waiting for the hormonal cues necessary to make its grand appearance. The layer of fat beneath baby's skin will continue to develop, aiding in temperature control outside the womb. Although baby may add a fraction of an inch to his overall length, most infants at this point already weigh a little over seven pounds, and measure around 20 inches—the size of a small watermelon. Boys may be slightly heavier than girls. The outer layers of baby's skin are sloughing off now, a process that will continue after birth, manifesting itself as dry, flaky skin. No special lotions or creams are needed, as a new layer of skin is already in the process of forming; it will be only a matter of time before baby's skin is as smooth as...well...a baby's bottom! At this point in development, even babies of a darker skin heritage will appear whitish, as their pigment has not yet fully developed. Baby's brain is continuing to grow in size, and will do so until about the third year of life.

What is Going On with Your Body at Thirty-Nine Weeks Pregnant?

At your weekly appointment, your practitioner will perform an internal exam, to determine whether any progress has been made in terms of dilation and effacement. Even if you are somewhat dilated, it is too early to uncork the champagne just yet, as it is entirely possible to walk around for weeks at the same dilation and effacement levels. On the other hand, it is also possible to have your first contraction shortly after your appointment, as labor could begin at literally any time now.

If you cannot possibly wait another day, let alone another week, to meet your precious baby, you can ask your OB/GYN, during the course of your internal exam, to strip your membranes. This simple procedure can be done if you are at least one centimeter dilated. Your OB/GYN will insert a finger into your cervix and separate the amniotic sac from the bottom of the uterus. This accomplishes two things. First, it weakens the amniotic sac (increasing its likelihood of breakage), and second, it aids in effacement (thinning) and dilation (opening) of your cervix. This perfectly safe and simple procedure may feel like a sharp pinch, and may lead to minimal spotting or cramping afterward, but having your membranes stripped is an excellent way to get the ball rolling without the harshness of labor-inducing agents such as Pitocin. Other natural methods, such as late-trimester sex, eating hot chilies, or bouncing on a trampoline may be fun to try, but there are no guarantees.

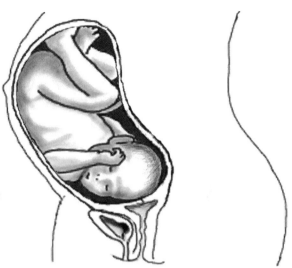

Now that you are forty weeks pregnant, the end is literally days away. If you have uneventfully passed your due date this week, chances are you are headed for an induction. Either way, your baby is coming VERY soon now, so enjoy what could be the final week of your pregnancy. What can you expect this week?

What is Going On with Your Baby at Forty Weeks Pregnant?

Babies vary in size depending upon their heritage, but the average newborn weighs around 7.5 pounds and measures about 20 inches long from head to heel. At this point, baby's skull bones are not yet fused, which enables the plates to semi-overlap as he or she exits the narrow birth canal. This may give your baby a charming "cone-headed" look when it is first born; this is entirely normal and temporary. This week, the placenta is providing baby with antibodies to stave off infections, a job that will be taken over by your breast milk once baby has entered the world. Baby has fattened up, and is officially ready to make his or her long-awaited debut into your loving arms.

When thinking about delivering a baby, many women wonder how something so big can possibly emerge from such a small opening. In reality, this condition, called cephalopelvic disproportion, should not be a concern for the majority of women for several reasons.

First of all, the pelvis is not a fixed structure. During the course of your pregnancy, the hormone relaxin has been hard at work loosening the ligaments that support the pelvic girdle, making it possible to accommodate your baby's head. Second of all, baby's skull is not yet fused, so the diameter of the head is also somewhat flexible. Thirdly, the position in which a woman delivers can make a huge difference in the ease of delivery. For instance, a squatting position can open the pelvic girdle up to 30% more than the typically employed semi-recline position. Finally, when it comes to genetics, most newborns are fairly well matched to the size of their mothers.

Your weight gain will have slowed, stopped, or even reversed by this week, as your pregnancy draws to a close. You may experience diarrhea this week as your body prepares for baby's arrival by making room any way it can. Some women also find themselves vomiting as labor begins.

Take comfort in the fact that all of the unpleasantness of pregnancy will soon be over, and chances are, you will not even remember most of it in the face of what you gain. Baby's movement slows down this week, as there is really no place left for it to go except out and down. Baby's head may be engaged already, making walking increasingly difficult as well as putting pressure on your bladder. Your practitioner will check for dilation and effacement at what could be your final appointment, and will listen to baby's heartbeat one more time. Know that the first stage of labor could take hours, and even days, so when that first contraction hits, remain calm, and call your practitioner to let him or her know that you will be on your way soon. The best of luck to you and your beautiful baby!

There you have it ladies. I hope that you liked my book, and that it was helpful. Enjoy your pregnancy and don´t worry too much. Life is a miracle!

Thanks for reading my book.

My very best,
Babette

www.whatoknowaboutpregnancy.co

Index

squatting position 98
stomach distress 79
stomach pain 63
Streptococcus bacteria 88
stretch marks 48
strip membranes 96
sweat glands 45
swelling 58, 63

T

taste buds 55
teeth 26
testicles 53, 66
third-trimester ultrasound 86
tooth buds 57
toxins 52
Trisomy-18 31

U

ultrasound 31, 43, 48
umbilical cord 22, 77
urinary tract infection 51
urination 21
urine 51
uterus 11, 14, 16, 21, 33, 51, 53, 54
UTI 51

V

vagina 12
varicose veins 43, 55
vernix caseosa 50, 85, 89
Vitamin B 11
vitamin C 74
vitamins 15
vocal cords 64

W

water 52, 54, 56
water breaking 63, 67, 92
weight gain 39, 71
wives' tales 58

X

X-rays 11

Y

yeast infections 51
yoga and Pilates 54
yolk sac 28

Notes

32220012R00061

Made in the USA
Middletown, DE
26 May 2016